MW00944069

From Wheels To Heals

A Chronic Pain Patients' Story of Hope, Help and Understanding

By Barby Ingle

Amazon bestselling author, reality television personality, and president of International Pain Foundation (iPain) sharing her powerful story about life-changing events that forced life reflection, purpose, and her journey from wheels to heals.

ISBN-13: 978-1542600194
ISBN-10: 1542600197
Copyright 2017
First Printing

From Wheels To Heals

A Chronic Pain Patients' Story of Hope, Help and Understanding

By Barby Ingle

Amazon bestselling author, reality television personality, and president of International Pain Foundation (iPain) sharing her powerful story about life-changing events that forced life reflection, purpose, and her journey from wheels to heals.

This book can be bought anywhere books are sold including Amazon Books, Barnes and Nobel, CreateSpace, Bookmans, Books-A-Million, Books, Inc., Deseret Books, Seagull Book, Follett's, Hudson News, Davis-Kidd Booksellers, LifeWay Christian Resources, Powell's Books, and Schuler Books & Music

ISBN-13: 978-1542600194
ISBN-10: 1542600197
Copyright 2017
First Printing

This book covers my story of the last 20 years of living with chronic pain diseases, learning to thrive despite the pain and my journey *From Wheels to Heals*. This book is written from the pain patient perspective, based on my experiences in dealing with pain and the healthcare system and what I have learned along the way.

In 1994, I earned a Bachelor of Science degree in social psychology from George Mason University. I then was a business owner of a successful cheerleading company – Cheertec and worked as a head cheerleading and dance coach at the Division IA Washington State University until my auto accident in 2002 force my retirement in July, 2003.

This book is intended to be a beacon of love, light, blessings, hope, and help. If you have medical questions, please research on your own outside of this book as well as speak with healthcare providers you trust. Every patient is different, we must find what is right for us individually. Just because it worked for me or others doesn't mean it is right for you. My hope is that the book does give you the motivation to become an engaged patient, because we all deserve proper and timely care.

This book is good for the chronically ill, pain patients, family members, caregivers, healthcare professionals and the public. One in three people in the United States are affected with a condition that causes pain, so it is bound to affect you or someone you know. Until you feel the pain, it is difficult to understand the challenges it brings on. Whether physical or mental, pain can, and will consume you if you allow it to.

Only the patient can begin the process of healing. My hope is that through my speaking engagements and books, I will inspire your eventual transformation of great positivity in life and one filled with hope. Healing starts from within. No pill or drug can duplicate the power within you. Here's to turning your pain to power!

INDEX

ENDO-WHAT?

Our long-term health and quality of life is important and would help all of society live better lives that are not as negatively impacted when chronic illnesses are suddenly part of what we live each day. I ask myself and providers why we are not taught about preventative health as children. Why are we not taught how the health system works until we must figure it out when a chronic illness is devastating our life and not before? I didn't even know that chronic illness could be a thing.

My mother was a Colonel in the US Army Stationed at Walter Reid Army Hospital, and President of the Virginia State Health Department Association and yet, I had no idea how the health system worked. The health system is there for acute conditions and catastrophic (when it meant death), but what about all the advances that have been made for those with chronic illnesses who don't die from what we face, but somehow get out of societies eye and mind with living daily and what that will mean for us.

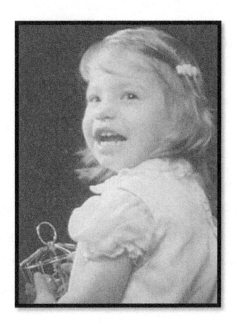

Baby Barby

Like many thousands of patients and caregivers I have talked to over the years, I was not prepared for life with chronic illness.

After college graduation in the summer of 1994, I moved to Washington State. My fiancé had moved there the year before me after his graduation to be closer to his biological father. The day I graduated, instead of attending the graduation ceremony,

I got on a plane and went to start my life with my soon to be husband. There was no reason to celebrate finishing school with this silly little walk across the stage ceremony. I did that in high school and it just held me up from getting to my first day at work at summer cheer camps with Eastern Cheerleaders Association.

Graduation was just an expectation in my family and the next step was 'adulting'. I packed everything I owned which was two duffle bags of clothes and some pageant trophies/crowns, and sashes. I left straight from my dorm room for the airport. My fiancé picked me up and took me to the apartment he had rented for us. It was next to a school. I had no idea what I was going to do or be. Night two my husband got home from work and after dinner we went for a walk. The cheerleaders at the school next to our apartments were out on the field practicing. They were horrible. I was so shocked. Coming from Virginia and competitive cheer teams and working for ECA I had seen peewee cheerleaders with more ability than this team. I wanted to go down and help them. Their coach needed help as well.

We went back to our apartment and talked about what we had just seen. The next day when he was at work I started planning and making goals. By the time, he came home, I had decided I was going to start my own cheerleading and dance training company. They obviously needed it there in WA state.

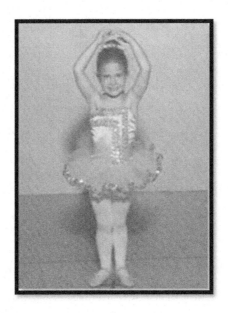

Ballet Barby

By the end of the week I started Western Cheerleading Association, had my business license and first set of flyers ready to send out to all the schools in the state. Within two weeks I had multiple schools book me for private training camps and the local parks and recreation office had asked me to teach a class on cheerleading once a week. The next month I married my husband and we were moving through life pretending to be adults that knew what we needed to know. You know how it is when you are 21, a college graduate, running a successful business and don't know that you should fear the societal boundaries that are all around us we just didn't know it.

In 1995, I heard from one of the cheer instructors I had hired that Washington State University was hiring their first spirit program coach. I of course applied and after interviews was offered the job. I could run both Cheertec and coach full time at WSU. It was a dream come true for me and I settled into a life I was very happy with.

WCA grew into what became a multi-state business with summer camps, cheer and dance competitions, and even teaching the state cheerleading coaches training program for all middle and high school coaches in the Northwestern states. Eventually we incorporated the company, upgraded the name to Cheertec, Inc., expanded out territory to the west coast, created a clothing line, and worked up to events with thousands in attendance and requiring large staffs.

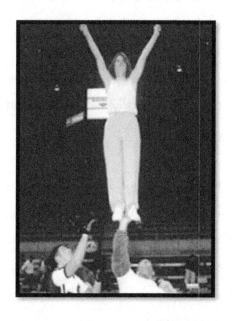

Barby in a Cheerleading Stunt

I had built a great life with my husband. I was taking life for granted. I had everything I ever wanted. In 1997 I began having pain in my lower abdomen which was worse with sex, lower back, pelvis and vagina. I began having abnormal menstruation and spotting. I also noticed severe constipation and nausea, feeling full all the time and cramping. Back in college I had multiple ovarian cysts and a miscarriage. I was told then that I was probably not going to be able to carry a baby to full term, but I never asked why. Now we found out.

Understanding that the cysts that I started developing in college were endometriosis induced ovarian cysts. I had endometriosis for years but ignored what I was going through until I couldn't. After seeing a gynecologist, taking medications, undergoing 6 months of Lupron shots that didn't help, undergoing a laparoscopy, counseling and the physical pain increasing I ended up going to a women's surgeon at the University of Washington. I was the youngest woman that the UW Women's Center had ever performed a full hysterectomy on. My doctor was amazing. She was very good, much better than the one I was seeing in Spokane. She and her team wanted to make sure that I understood that even though I knew I didn't want a baby and chance of being able to have one were slim after a full hysterectomy I would not be able to have one for sure. I totally understood. I was also tired of not having pain free days. I wanted my pain free life back. If it took this type of major surgery to get it, that was fine with me. December 1999, I underwent the surgery. My dad, brother, husband and in-laws were all there with me. They took great care of me. It was a long 3-month recovery. I was so excited to be back and living with no pain, no drain, no problems. Life was grand, I was back to coaching and best of all, pain-free. I felt like if I could make it through this, I could make it through anything.

For most of the first 29 years of my life, I got to live out all my dreams. If I dreamed it, I worked hard to create it. I took life for granted in so many ways though. I didn't realize how fragile it is and how much our daily health really mattered. Although my marriage started having trouble in early 2002, I found out that my husband had cheated on me one day when he collapsed and was taken to the emergency room. He had thyroid cancer back in 1993 and here we were in 2002 and he had a complication with his thyroid levels. I thought I would be a good wife and help him out with his email when I found some that alarmed me. When he got home we talked it out and he admitted to me that he did in fact cheat. I was dedicated to making my marriage work not only because that was what I was supposed to do but because I am Catholic and it was against my religion. I started counseling. I was religious but my husband was not. I was working full time and running Cheertec and he had just started working part time that year. I wanted to go to counseling, he didn't believe in it. So, I went alone in hopes of saving my marriage.

About a month later I was on my way into work and an 8 second minor auto accident changed my life once again.

TRY HARDER

When I became so debilitated by the pain and doctors could not figure out what was going on, I could no longer hold my life together. It was a minor auto accident that was causing crazy symptoms that didn't make sense to me or the providers I was going to.

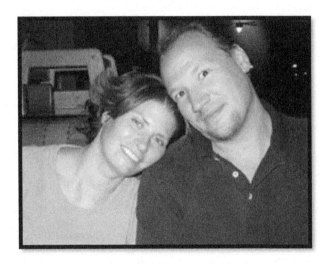

Barby and Ken (her husband)

When my symptoms first began, I thought I was being ridiculous. The pain was overwhelming. It took my attention, my energy, my ability to focus. It was a burning fire pain in my face, neck and shoulder, skin discoloration. I started having balance issues and falling. I remember at one practice I was working with a male cheerleader and we did a stunt. Everyone around us was yelling, "Coach, stand up straight, what are you doing?". I kept saying I was straight. I finally looked down. I don't even know how he was holding me up in the air. I was in the weirdest position, legs bent, leaning forward, arms not in the right place. Until I looked down and saw what my body was doing I had no idea what everyone was upset about.

I was now coaching, heading to counseling appointments, chiropractics, neurologists and sleeping in my office or where ever I could find a place to sleep. I would sleep unless I had to be awake for my job. I was overwhelmed physically and emotionally. Not being able to coach, but still trying I know I let my team members down that year. I wish I could go back and help them understand what I was going through. I wish I had let go of my job sooner so that they could have had a better year. I didn't know that what I was dealing with was not going to be as easily overcome as endometriosis was. And that was a struggle that made me believe everything was just a challenge that I could get past. Not this time, it was going to take years, millions of dollars, and learning new life skills. I just didn't know it.

I was no longer able to do my dream job; coaching cheer and dance at a division I-A University. My business started to crumble and eventually closed. My marriage fell apart and my husband stopped supporting me emotionally and physically. I didn't have the energy to take care of me and him any longer. One good thing that came from it was after our separation he found God, and was baptized into the Catholic church the next Easter.

The biggest reason it fell apart was he had me feeling that it was all in my head and tried to convince my family and our friends of the same. My psychologist and psychiatrist both decidedly told me my ex-husband was wrong. I was diagnosed with situational depression. They assured me that what I was going through was normal for what I was going through. They had faith in me and helped me get faith back in myself.

While my ex-husband tried to say, I was bipolar because I no longer could hold 'us' together and had to focus on making sure I was going to be okay. The only thing was that I knew for sure from the moment of the accident was that I would not do this to myself. I didn't understand it, but I fought moment by moment to keep living the best I could. I had begun marriage counseling before the accident because of our struggling relationship, now that was no longer an issue because the relationship was over. We were divorced within 3 months of filing for separation. Now I needed help getting my new life in order and continued counselling until I felt I had the life tools I needed to be the best me I could be.

I rated the physical pain I had from the accident in the beginning as a level ten. I did not think I could take anything worse. As each surgery or procedure was performed and the pain worsened, I realized that I wish I had that first pain back if I had to have pain at all. As our bodies get "used to the pain", the pain is easier to manage and deal with. With each additional trauma and spread of the reflex sympathetic dystrophy, the pain you thought was unbearable becomes an okay level.

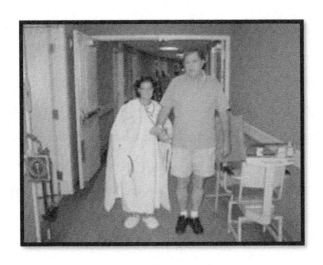

Barby and Her Dad

Reflex Sympathetic Dystrophy has undergone over 20 name changes over the years. It will continue to do so, but I was diagnosed with RSD eventually. Reflex is any process in your body that is automatic going haywire. Sympathetic is your sympathetic nervous system, and dystrophy is loss of muscle and bone. As an athlete, it was difficult to understand how working out and pushing myself was making me worse, it was.

CHANGE IN FAMILY DYNAMICS

Chronic pain can involve a lifelong condition that has a significant impact not only on the patient but on family and friends as well. The condition may affect many aspects of the patient's life in varying degrees including activities of daily living, professional, social and personal life. The patient must make some adjustments. After health, patients are usually hit hardest in the financial aspects of this chronic disorder. They frequently need a leave of absence from work or possibly early retirement due to inability or difficulty performing work-related tasks. With less money and mobility, they tend to give up or modify leisure activities such as hiking, kayaking, traveling, and participating in family activities and outings. Exercising becomes difficult, if not impossible, to manage. Everyday activities such as driving and shopping must be given up or modified. Financial difficulties are acerbated due to frequent visits to health-care providers, medical-related expenses and unemployment.

Friends and family may find it beneficial to map out a plan of action with the patient's participation so that a daily routine is established. This reduces stress levels and minimizes unexpected changes in plans. Responsibilities that may need to be addressed include:

- Car pools
- Chores/housework
- Cooking
- Holiday activities
- Jobs (employment)
- Laundry
- Leisure activities
- Pet care
- Planning meals
- Self-care
- Sex life
- Shopping
- Social life

The patient should be encouraged to stay active and to join a support group or seek psychological counseling if appropriate. Patients may even reach the point of ultimately counseling others with chronic pain. Some patients find benefit in getting involved in volunteer work, which allows them to set their own hours and to feel that they still can contribute to others instead of just focusing on their own condition.

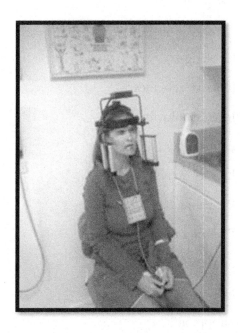

Barby Going Through Diagnostic Testing

Despite a wide range of treatment options available to patients with chronic pain, some patients do not seek help since they may be discouraged by constant pain and are worn down both physically and emotionally. This may result in their dismissing efforts by others to help them.

Some of their concerns include:

- Fear of side effects from treatments
- Fear that nothing can help them
- Fear that they will be a "complainer" if they talk about their pain
- Fear that they will become addicted to medications
- Fear that they will develop a tolerance to medications and the recurring pain will be even worse

It is important to discuss these concerns with family members, friends, physicians, or support service professionals (e.g., psychologist, social worker), to take advantage of options that are available and may lead to pain relief and improvement in the overall quality of life. I can see how it is difficult (or impossible) to imagine that someone can be in severe pain continually if one has not experienced it. It is normal for you not to understand it if you have not lived through it. I did not understand and as a former athlete, it was hard to talk about pain and what I was going through. Society also does not often address the issues around chronic pain either. I often hear "you look healthy," but often I suffer excruciating, unforgiving, and burning pain.

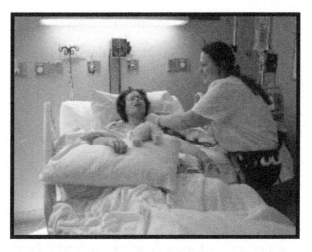

Barby in hospital after TOS surgery

For a caretaker, it may be hard to stand by and accept that your loved one's pain cannot be fixed or cured (although it may be eased). It may also be hard to accept that you cannot make it better. If you are in a close relationship with someone with chronic pain, you are likely to develop a variety of negative feelings as a result. This is a normal part of the process. Your emotions can range from anger to resentment. Both you and the loved one in pain are victims of the pain problem. Significant lifestyle changes will affect the caretaker; for instance: time, social support, outside intrusions, and reduced income.

- Anxiety and guilt due to financial problems that result from your loved one's disability and the realization you can't help cure them
- Because of a withdrawal of affection or a decline in your sex life, you may develop depression.
- You get angry if the person is irritable or withdrawn.
- You may become resentful having to take over tasks they previously performed.
- You take on stress because of others' reactions. For example, "he doesn't look that disabled to me" or "why doesn't he want to work?"

Family and friends often become caretakers for the patient in pain and are also victims of the pain problem. Both patients and caretakers experience reduced social support and intrusions into your life. For example, some insurance companies may follow or film you and your families, thinking that you are all in on faking for financial gain.

Your family may have a reduction of income or must work harder to stay afloat financially to make up for the lost wages of the patient. Due to reduced income, unemployment, and medical expenses required for various treatments, family income can be cut in half or diminish to nothing. It may be shrewd for the patient and their family to meet with a financial planner or an insurance agent and devise a budget so that future and unexpected expenses will be accounted for. This may reduce the general stress level for the patient and their loved ones.

This can become a harsh reality. I lost my job and had no income of my own. My family and caretakers had to help me out or I would become indigent. Until my social security disability kicked in, I was basically at the mercy of food stamps and family support. It is not only financially hard on direct family; often time extended family is asked to step in and help. If they cannot see the injury or they do not believe the patient in pain, it becomes very difficult. I have undergone significant lifestyle changes. I used to be able to do things like eating out often, cooking, shopping, driving, and cleaning. These activities are now challenges, both financially and physically. Again, turning to family and friends as caretakers and support outlets is important for the patient.

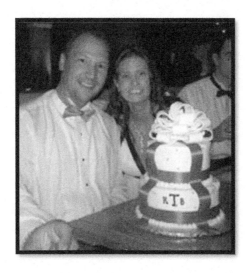

Ken and Barby Enjoying Their Wedding Reception

Remember, caretakers are also going through life changes because of supporting the patient. They now must take time getting you to medical or other appointments if you cannot drive. They may end up doing most or all household chores and child-rearing activities. Understanding that this is hard on you and your caretakers is important for better communication. Caretakers may also experience some positive outcomes, although this is less common. If you were controlling, they may have to accept that they have more freedom, or if they have a very strong need to help others, they may feel good about helping you.

To have the caretakers take care of themselves first is most important. You cannot take care of someone else properly if you are not keeping yourself together. Try not to feel guilty when you need a break to do something for you. No one can be there for someone else around the clock. You can take care of yourself by choosing a healthy lifestyle that puts yourself first.

When it comes to communication with the patient, try to avoid hurtful comments like, "you'll just have to live with it." Pay attention to your gestures and non-verbal communication. Rejection shows through actions as well as words. How you choose to say something, your tone of voice, facial expressions, and eye contact, or lack of, are all signs of rejection, resentment and show other negative feelings. When you see someone frowning or sneering they do not have to say a word and you can guess well what is going through their mind. Your gestures communicate just as much as words do.

Communication with your family member in pain is a family challenge, not just an individual one. Try to see the disability as a challenge that you all face together. Take the approach of "we," not "he," will fight this together. Listening to what the patient is saying and watching what you say can keep the lines of communication open. Pretending to be interested when you are not can create a breakdown in communication and in your ability to help the other person and vice versa.

Be real with your emotions. If you do not believe, ask more questions, and get more information. It matters that you accept their pain to be as they say it is. Do not tell them "it can't be that bad" unless you are trying to hurt them and the situation. If you pay attention not only to what your loved one is saying, but to their nonverbal communication and how they are saying it, they may be less reluctant to talk about how they feel or give indications in their behavior as to how they are doing. If you have questions about your patient's pain reports, remember that chronic pain is rarely imaginary.

You may question if they could be faking it to get out of work or some other challenge. Consciously faking pain to get out of something or to get a reward is known as malingering. While it does occur, it is rare. Most patients will feel very guilty about not being able to do the things they used to do, whether working at a job or doing chores around the house. Negative emotions from the patient or to the patient such as depressed mood, anger, or anxiety play an important role in increasing pain levels. When confronted with these emotions, be sure to recognize them but don't take them personally. For the patient, anxiety, stress and anger can cause an increase in muscle tension leading to more pain.

I am most helped in my chronic pain when those closest to me express concern for my suffering and offer help that is genuinely needed. Their encouragement for me to be as active as possible helps me stay social through rough days. As a caretaker, do not overdo your sympathy or try to remove all obstacles and challenges from someone in pain. On the other hand, do not punish the sufferer through blame and hostility. If you are not sure how best to be helpful, you might ask the person in pain what kind of attention they feel is most helpful and respectful. Judging how the patient is doing without asking them is going to be based on your perception and may not be accurate. Remember, people in pain learn coping skills as time goes on, and they may not be crying all the time but still have severe pain.

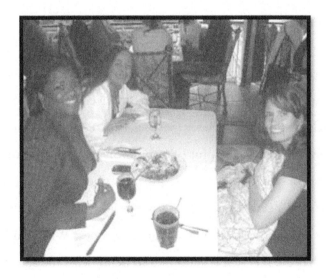

Barby, Her Mom and Sister out to lunch

It is also helpful to me when people close to me show encouragement when I am trying to be as active as possible. I can tell when people are overdoing sympathy. I like to challenge myself but find that some people will try to remove all obstacles and challenges from me because I am in pain. On the other hand, I do not like being punished by blame and hostility when I can do something at a good moment and need help with the same task later. I like when people ask me what kind of attention and assistance I need. It feels helpful and respectful and puts me at ease.

My husband attends medical visits with me. When attending medical visits with me, he gets involved in the conversation when appropriate. Since meeting, before we even dated, he has only missed a handful of appointments. I have him ask the doctor what medications are prescribed, dosages, and how often I need to take them. I have had trouble in the past with overdosing or missing medication at times. With him knowing what the regimen is supposed to be, it helps me stay on track. When he understands, what medication is prescribed and the overall treatment plan, he can better understand what I am going through. Also, chronic pain patients and pain patients in general, have trouble with short-term memory. This is caused by multiple factors. The sleep cycle is disturbed causing a lack of concentration. The medications they take make them groggy or less able to concentrate. For me, the biggest reason is that the pain is overwhelming. It is hard to concentrate when pain levels are high.

Having your caretaker taking notes at the doctor's office can remind them and the patient of important information about new medications, research to do, and approved activities. When I was in physical therapy, my husband asked questions and then worked with the PT on me to be able to perform traction and massage at home properly.

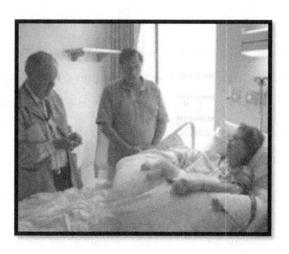

Barby, Her Father, and Priest at a Hospital Visit

The healthcare provider and physical therapist can also help you understand what the appropriate level of activity is for your loved one. It is important to find the boundary between motivation and hurtful nudge. It is important to understand the overall treatment plan and help the pain patient stick to it. I have seen firsthand that dealing with severe pain can be overwhelming for both the patients and those who care for them. Working together with everyone involved will take some of the stress and anxiety off everyone. Try to be an advocate for your patient. Going to the doctor with a hidden agenda can make matters worse. For example, some people ask the doctor who prescribes the medications if he thinks they are necessary to undermine his authority. This type of attitude affects how the doctor sees the patient on a treatment level. Also, both the doctor and the patient can become isolated from you.

My mother worked in the healthcare industry until her recent retirement. She attended a doctor's appointment with me in Colorado and was with me during my first rib surgery in Arizona. She knows enough to try to help me, but in speaking up in the tone and manner with which she approached the doctors got to them. One even wrote a note in my records. The entire time I was in another surgery, my mother told my husband she had a bad feeling that things were done incorrectly by the doctors, all before I even got out of surgery. This scares the hell out of anyone. It is important to be positive about these situations once the decision is made to go forward. In the end, I did have complications on that surgery, but there is a better way to handle a stressful medical situation and a better way to approach the doctors. On the next surgery, I took my husband and my father, who also asked questions, but were there to support me in a positive manner. The doctor was much more receptive in sharing information and showed a genuine will to help. The problem is not asking questions; it is trying to meet your own agenda that breaks down patient and doctor communications. Advocating for your patient requires tact, unless of course they are in a dangerous situation.

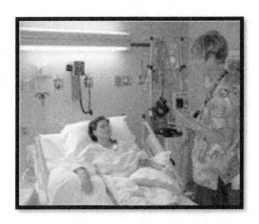

Barby and Her Nurse at a Hospital Visit

One study evaluating quality of life issues among patients with chronic pain reported that the greatest interruption in daily life was related to activities of living.[1] The greatest disruptions in my daily life are directly related to pain, difficulty sleeping, and lack of energy. In the beginning, mobility was not a significant

---

[1] Health-Related Quality of Life in Chronic Refractory Reflex Sympathetic Dystrophy (Complex Regional Pain Syndrome Type I). Journal of Pain and Symptom Management, Volume 20, Issue 1, Pages 68 – 76, M. Kemler

issue for me, but in 2006 I began having chronic pain symptoms in my foot and began having problems with a greater range of symptoms. It increased the amount of coping needed to accomplish my daily activities.

Family and friends who form the support group around the patient must be educated and aware about chronic pain, its treatment and rehabilitation, behaviors of the patient that should be encouraged or discouraged, and supporting roles they can play. It is very important for friends and family to understand what the patient is going through and allow the patient the opportunity to express his or her grief and frustration without being judgmental. Family and friends also need to be supportive and to encourage the patient to keep his or her spirits up and to continue functioning to the best of his or her ability. Some patients become depressed if their condition prevents them from doing things that are important to their independence and well-being. Formerly independent people may have to rely on others for daily tasks (e.g., dressing, cooking, and errands). Having to have someone assist you is inconvenient and can make you feel you have a loss of self-respect. It is important to address these feelings and to respond appropriately.

WERE GOING SOMEWHERE

My treatment plan from 2005 to 2009 is having a radiofrequency (RF) procedure on a 5-6-week basis, and I receive a sympathetic nerve block (SNB) along with my RF treatment through which I get relief. Although not all my symptoms or pain goes away, the relief is priceless. Other people experience pain relief from just a SNB depending upon the severity of the chronic pain. The SNB does not block motor activity so you can remain mobile and active which offers you better range of motion. Your range of motion and exercises can increase during the time the nerve block has reduced the degree of pain.

My doctor also cautions me every time about the risks in undergoing the RF. Risks include new nerve injuries, bleeding, allergic reactions to the medications being used, seizures, and the stress and fear about the procedure. It is important that you have a competent pain management specialist because of the variety of complications involved in performing the procedure. My pain specialist happens to be an anesthesiologist who is experienced with the RF technique and is comfortable performing it on me. I suggest that you only get a RF procedure from a trained professional who treats chronic pain patients specifically and has performed this procedure on a regular basis. I have other symptoms after my procedure that my doctor reports are not common. It is important to notify your doctor of any side affects you may have or complications noted after the procedure. Further complications may develop or become life threatening if not taken care of when they first begin. After the procedure, I have a low-grade fever, stiff neck, general achiness for up to seven days, and basic flu like symptoms before the pain decreases.

Some doctors will try to go from a successful SNB or RF to a chemical or surgical Sympathectomy. A Sympathectomy involves cutting out the sympathetic ganglion nerve bundle, which is in a specific area along the spinal cord. Once the nerve bundle is removed, there is nothing for the doctor to treat if the pain returns. Sympathectomy is a procedure that has high risks, and the outcome varies from patient to patient; this should be used as a last resort. Carefully weigh the risks of the procedure and communicate with your doctor in detail.

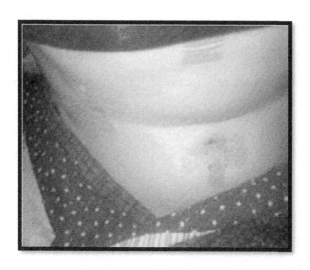

Barby's Bandages After Gall Bladder Surgery

If it is determined that the source of the chronic pain is sympathetically maintained, in which pain is reduced with a sympathetic nerve block (SNB), then this may be an option. However, if the pain is determined to be sympathetically independent pain, a Sympathectomy is not a procedure that will benefit you. Once performed, the removal is permanent. Even if you have SMP, it may turn into SIP down the road with the additional trauma to the body, so the risks of failure are high for this procedure. If you have chosen to receive a full Sympathectomy, you will be limited or out of treatment options. With the possible risks, make sure that you are an appropriate candidate for this procedure and that you are willing to undergo the procedure despite the risks. Remember, this procedure does not always work even when the chronic pain is sympathetically driven.

The procedure that I received every six weeks, radio-frequency ablation, is technically considered a Sympathectomy. The radiofrequency (RF) ablation uses radio-frequency heat to collapse veins around nerve tissue, which decreases pain signals and allows me to experience partial relief.

My high pain levels return after four to six weeks as the nerves reawaken. Patients may have complete relief or no relief at all. Although most patients do experience complete or partial relief for several months, the effects are not lasting. The burning pain during this time is reduced for me after those few days of flu-like symptoms. Only a small percent (15-30%) experience long-term relief lasting two years or longer.

In a study published in 2002 in the Journal of Vascular Surgery, researchers from the University of South Florida College of

Medicine reported that patients had at least 50% reduction in pain intensity after a Sympathectomy. Only a small percent of patients reported no relief at all and are considered treatment failures.[2]

The post Radiofrequency pain and sickness I experienced was associated with the surgical aspects of the procedure, which has been reported to occur in about 40% of patients. Other symptoms I notice after my procedure are excessive sweating, increase in my Horner's syndrome and extremely low blood pressure after the procedure is finished. Horner's syndrome is a syndrome caused by injury to the sympathetic nerves of the face, which includes a constricted pupil, drooping eyelids, and facial dryness. Below is a picture of me when my Horner's Syndrome was very apparent.

Other patients have also reported post Radiofrequency symptoms like pneumothorax, seizures and a recurrence or worsening of the chronic pain. Be sure to find a surgeon with

---

[2] Journal of Vascular Surgery, researchers from the University of South Florida College of Medicine

experience and a high success rate with any of the sympathectomy procedures before you schedule one for yourself.

An additional option is the use of a tens unit, which is also known as a nerve stimulator. The tens unit provides electrical nerve stimulation that, in small amounts to the nerves, overcomes the sensation of pain. It is a trick to your nerves. Think about when you have hurt yourself on something in the past. Your reaction is to rub the area. This causes a good sensation to be sent to the brain, which can sometimes help forget the pain. This does not always work, but the tens unit has been beneficial to me. I use the tens unit because it is non-invasive. Mine is battery-operated, portable and available for self-treatment because it is a small unit. I can use it as needed and can place the electrodes where I need them most. Although I have not experienced negative effects from the tens unit, some people get skin rashes from the sticky side of the electrode. Also, people with pacemakers and pregnant women should not use the tens unit or the spinal cord stimulator.

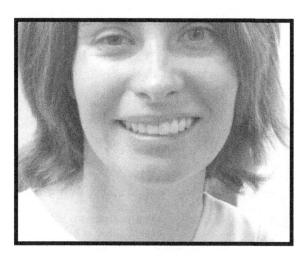

Horner's Syndrome is Evident in the Right Eye, an Indication of Neurological Damage

Other treatment options for chronic pain patients include topical pain patches; I use Lidoderm patches as well as lidocaine lotion. Other topical medications used are fontanel and clonidine. Be sure to check with your doctor about potential side effects. Some chronic pain patients also use acupuncture as a treatment. I am weary of this because any trauma to the body can increase your symptoms and cause additional problems. Other adverse issues with acupuncture include: bleeding, inflammation, intensification of pain, nerve irritation and or injury, infections, poor wound healing, and skin irritations.

The good news is that no matter how long you have had chronic pain you can be helped in some way, if you are willing to stay active, can avoid surgical procedures, can change medication usage when needed and will improve eating habits. Unfortunately, chronic pain affects many systems of the body over time, the autonomic and central nervous system, immune system, limbic, gastrointestinal and more. Patients can convince themselves that a doctor or surgeon can perform surgery on them that will cure them. In the beginning, I was one of these patients myself.

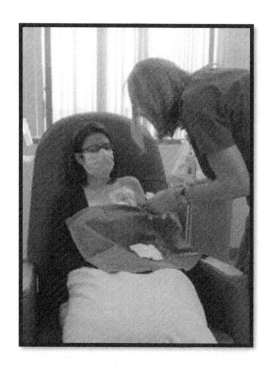

Barby and Her Infusion Nurse

Resorting to surgery can lead a chronic pain patient to a wheelchair and the need for larger doses of narcotic medication at an accelerated rate. As of now, there is no quick fix for chronic pain. There is not even a great treatment method that works for all patients. In 1983, Dr. Poplawski from Canada published a study about the outcome of chronic pain. He showed that chronic pain diagnosed in the first two years has a chance of successful treatment in 80% of the patients, and after two years, each year drops the percentage of the success significantly.[3] other doctors' say within the first six to nine months is the window for remission.

I consider these milestones as successful treatment of chronic pain:

- Ability to achieve a full night's sleep repeatedly
- Ability to perform physical therapy with marked improvement in muscle strength
- Decreased need for opioids
- Diminished depression
- Diminished swelling of the effected arm or leg
- Improved thinking
- Increased stamina
- Lowered pain levels, or pain controlled with low to moderate consideration

---

[3] Poplawski ZJ, Wiley AM, Murray JF: Post traumatic dystrophy of the extremities. J Bone Joint Surg [Am] 1983; 65:642-55

PEOPLE IN YOUR LIFE

Creating a support system in your life is a must! Your support system can take the form of your family, friends, a support group, healthcare providers, and caretakers. You may find it beneficial to map out a plan of action with your support team so that a daily routine is established and maintained. This can serve to minimize stress levels when unexpected changes in plans arise.

When you have chronic pain, making life as stress free as possible is important. Of course, you are changing inside. As you change physically and mentally, the people around you must also adjust. As they do, you may find that they do not fit into your life the same way or at all. Some people cannot handle watching someone else in pain and feel bad that they cannot fix it. They may tend to react by cutting you off or ignoring you. They may also compensate by bullying you or babying you.

The reality of your new situation is that as the change is taking place on the inside, you must also deal with the outside. You can make positive changes with dealing and communicating with others in your life and the new roles assumed by you and them. Transforming our world so that our most precious resources on the inside work together with our outer influences will help us with our new daily reality.

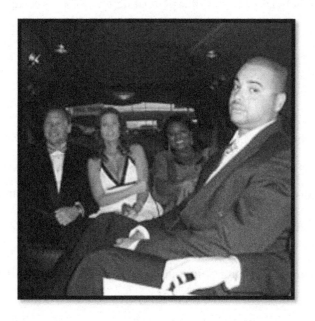

Barby, Ken And Her Family

Changing your approach to situations and your perspective makes you see things from a different angle. You can prepare and react to the new roles that those around you take on. Learning to use the people in your life to better your situation will also help them stay positive, and they can play larger roles in your life, whether it means backing off from some people or embracing offers from others. Limiting your time, discussions or interactions with people in your life will help everyone cope with stress of your new disability.

Look at your life as different, not over. Try arousing your hidden inner potential by trying new activities, learning new subjects and working to create balance and harmony between how you feel and what you can do. Bring out the good qualities that you have hidden inside you by experiencing the freedom of being your genuine self. When you're in pain it is hard to be anything but your true self; it can expose the raw side of who you are. The pain has helped me gain self-knowledge, avoid unnecessary detours in life and cultivate love and goodness in myself and in those I, choose to have around me. By my learning to manage pain, fear and anger, I have been able to create new circumstances and enjoy a better life quality, allowing those around me to also become better people. Paying attention to how you are living and reacting has many positive advantages. It has helped me become the person I want to be towards others in my life as well as become more spiritual. It has been helpful in refining my values. Living in pain has given me the chance to experience real satisfaction and happiness, forgive myself, and love and embrace myself on a grand level.

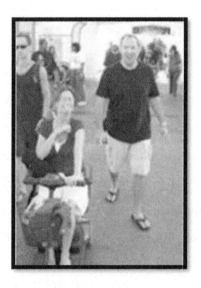

Barby and Ken on Their Honeymoon

How can you take the step in using those in your life to assist you, without taking advantage of them? Start with making a list of what needs to be done. Decide what you can do on the list and what you need assistance with. Responsibilities that need to be considered include: cleaning, cooking, laundry, mail drop off and delivery, pet care, planning meals, shopping, social activities and transportation.

Below are tips to accomplish tasks of daily living.

Cleaning

- Ask others to assist with the heavy work such as vacuuming and mopping.
- Choose one room every few days to concentrate on picking up or dusting.
- Hire a cleaning service.
- Put items away as you use them.
- Transportation
- Bring extra medication with you in case you have a flare up.
- Double check times, dates and locations of appointments before you leave the house.
- Use pillows and blankets to stay warm and comfortable.
- Shopping
- Have a plan as to what you are looking for and what

you want to accomplish while you are out.

- Use assistive devices that allow you to use less energy so you're able to shop longer.

Cooking

- Have someone cut food for you (or buy precut food), store in small containers for easy use when needed.
- Make small meals.
- Split up larger items into small, more manageable containers.

Laundry

- Have someone assist with folding, ironing and putting away the clothes.
- Sort laundry as it is dirtied (whites, colors, to be dry-cleaned).
- Wash more frequently.
- Wash smaller loads.

Planning Meals

- Choose items easy to make.
- Choose items that have a longer shelf life.
- Keep items on lower shelves.
- Order items from stores with home delivery.

Pet Care

- Ask neighborhood kids to take the dog for a walk or play with him in the park.
- Install a doggie door.
- Use larger food bowls so that they do not need to be filled as often.

Mail Drop off and Delivery

- Prepare your bills and outgoing mail so that next time you go out or someone comes to visit, it is ready to go and easily dealt with.
- The delivery guy can carry the items into your house instead of dropping them on the porch

Social Activities

- Choose creative activities you enjoy and are less physically demanding.
- Let the people attending know that you have good and bad days or moments and you may not be able to make it, may leave early or come late.
- Let them know ahead of time if you need quiet space.
- Let them know how you want to be greeted such as a

hug, air hug, hand shake, or head nod.

WHAT BROUGHT ME TO WHEELS?

Did I have something wrong with me physically? Was it in my head? With more pain, vision difficulties, doctors, blackouts, memory trouble and so on, the worse my life became. I began taking depression and anxiety medication on a regular basis. I really did not know what to think anymore; who was I? I asked everyone around me what they thought I should do. I no longer trusted what my body was telling me. I tried to convince myself that things were in my head and that I was strong enough to get over the pain and other symptoms on my own. I thought I just needed to try harder.

I constantly questioned my actions and stopped trusting my instincts. Through counseling, I got my voice back, renewed my confidence, found who I am, and what I am made of. This all helped me face the fact that this pain is a new reality for me, but I was going to find a way to LIVE. I went to a compassionate doctor, Dr. French, in Washington State, which was where I was living at the time. After he did his poking and prodding on me, he diagnosed me with a brachia plexus shoulder injury. It was then recommended to me to get doctors that were more specialized.

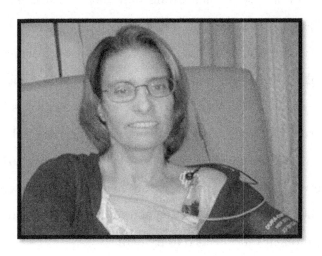

Barby at an Infusion Procedure

Some of my healthcare professionals in Washington found a doctor and physical therapist in Arizona that specialized in athletic injuries. Since I was an athlete, this made sense to me. This Arizona doctor would help me get back to the athletic state I was at physically prior to the accident. Thinking that it was a good idea, and after losing my job and barely hanging onto my marriage, we packed up and moved to Arizona. The day I arrived in AZ, I started physical therapy. A month later,

I was going into surgery to fix my shoulder and finally stop the pain. Even though the MRI and X-rays showed there was no injury, the doctor thought it would be best to go through with the surgery. At that point, I was ready for anything that would stop the pain. After surgery, the pain was not gone, and symptoms became worse. I realized that there is more than one type of physical pain and I was experiencing many of them at the same time. I continued to see more doctors; they were ruling out everything but could not tell me what was wrong.

Finally, I found a neurologist who had some new tests for me to undergo. They came back showing that I now had Thoracic Outlet Syndrome (TOS) and that there was a way to fix it. It would just be one more surgery by a vascular surgeon. The vascular surgeon performed his own vascular study/tests and confirmed the diagnosis. A week later, I was having my first rib removed. This surgery was a lot more complicated and had many risks. At this point, I was separated from my husband and did not know anyone in Arizona to help me except doctors. I began paying a neighbor to drive me to appointments and assist me with daily activities around my house.

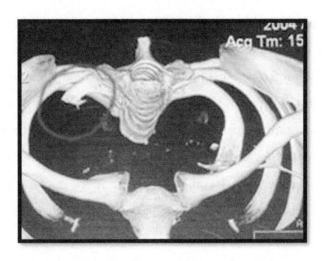

A picture from the 3-D body scan of patient Barby Ingle shows the two spurs on the right first rib after removal. One spur went into the right lung and the other was hooked into the right Brachia Nerve Bundle. The spurs resulted in the need for a repeat of the right first rib resection surgery.

Putting my trust in this new person, the only person willing to take care of me (though for a price), I decided to go through with the surgery. This surgery was going to be my miracle. After the surgery, I tried to convince myself that I was all better. And some things were better; I was not so tired. But overall, I was worse off than before, and with new symptoms, life became much harder. I thought the original pain was bad, but at that point, I thought if I had to have pain, I wanted the first pain back. On top of the pain, I now had a problem with my right lung. After five lung collapses, some requiring hospital stays, as well as an additional emergency lung procedure, I was turned over to new doctors who checked out my lung and could not understand why I was developing pneumothoraxes.

After two months, I went back to the neurologist. My symptoms were worse, and I passed out in his office while he was touching, poking, pulling and examining me. He realized that there was still a major problem and sent me to a doctor in Colorado. Dr. Brantigan was also a vascular surgeon, but he was one of the doctors who had perfected the TOS surgery. He ran a 3-D body scan and found that the first vascular doctor did a poor job. I had bone spurs, one going into my lung and one going into my nerve bundle. No wonder things were getting worse. I already had a pain in my nerves and the TOS surgery just increased the problem. So, my hope was raised once again. I was going to get one more surgery and be back to my old life.

By this time, I was devastated financially and could no longer pay my neighbor. Luckily, he was intrigued with something he saw in me. He also thought, "Anytime now, she is going to be fine." He moved in with me to take care of me full time. Since I could not pay him, this worked out perfectly. Spending so much time with the only person in AZ I knew who was not a doctor or lawyer, I began to have feelings for him, and we began to date, if you can call it that. I did not get out much.

After this latest surgery, I went into physical therapy again. I had a new PT, and he treated me as if I was a healthy athlete and pushed me through our sessions. EVERY session, I would leave in severe pain, crying, dizzy, walking into walls and to the point of vomiting. He said he was waiting for me to have a breakthrough. He told me my nerve was stuck and to just keep pushing with the weights and one day it would just pop free! I was getting worse and my drill sergeant of a physical therapist was making it worse. He also could not understand how, although I was hurting so badly, I would not put ice on after my sessions. That would have just been adding insult to my injuries. The ice was excruciating. I had a knee surgery in 2001 where I used ice after surgery to keep the swelling down and I loved it. However, this time the ice was bad, but I did not know why since it worked so well with my knee in the past.

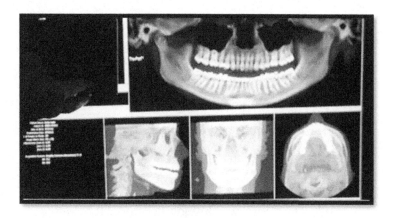

X-ray of Barby's Jaw

One day, my PT was out of town on business. I was very scared but went with a different therapist from the same office for the week. For once, I was in good hands. Paul, my substitute PT, began by asking me questions. He asked me things about my everyday life (activities of daily living), my symptoms and said he wanted to try a different approach. I was scared but wanted to do anything to get better. He took away all the weights and machines and began traction and a bit of nerve stretching. The traction was the greatest thing I had experienced in a long time, but the nerve stretching was still excruciating.

Each time he stretched me, he went right back to the traction, which brought the pain level down. This was great; I was finally able to get my arm into a semi-straight position. This was relief from the curled-up limb I was used to by then. I worked with Paul for five months and never went back to my old PT. Paul's specialty was treating patients with chronic pain such as TOS and RSD. We would talk about the symptoms and I began to consider it on my own through the internet resources I could find. So many people were in the same situation as I was, going from doctor to doctor with little to no relief, having a weird collection of symptoms that did not make sense to any of the doctors who saw them.

When I went back to my neurologist for a checkup, I brought what I had printed off the internet about RSD and pointed out to him that I thought I had this horrible condition. He assured me that I did not have RSD, and he was "100 percent sure". He decided to refer me to a pain specialist to get a shot of cortisone, also known as a trigger point injection. He also referred me to a plastic surgeon, as I have large breasts and he thought that much of my pain could be coming from my breast size as well. I saw the plastic surgeon and pain specialists on the same day. I didn't mention RSD to either of the new providers. This was my #41 and #42 in the new provider count. The pain management doctor suggested I schedule a TPI as soon as possible and the plastic surgeon said that she could remove my breasts but she didn't think that was the problem. She suggested a new doctor. Turned out to be the best referral of them all, #43.

FINDING MY PROVIDERS

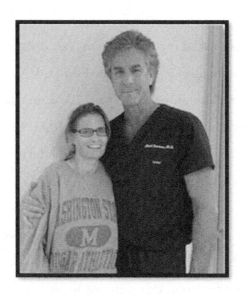

Barby with Dr. Mark Berman of Stem Cell Revelation

After all this time, I had finally found him: the doctor who knew. The pain specialist seemed as knowledgeable as Paul and was caring and willing to help. Dr. Rubin listened to me, evaluated me and then put everything together. He thought I might have RSD. He wanted to run a test and it involved a needle. At this point, after going through more EMGs than was reasonable for medical treatment, I was reluctant. I also pointed out that my previous doctor said he was 100 percent sure that I did not have reflex sympathetic dystrophy.

Dr. Rubin asked me what test my last doctor had performed to determine this. I told him the list of test and surgeries that I had been through over the past 2.5 years. He explained that none of those tests would show RSD and that this test wouldn't be pleasant but would help if I did have RSD. I placed my trust and pain in his hands.

A week later, I had the test. I did not expect any relief. A miracle happened; within 15 minutes of the procedure, I could straighten my arm. Although not all the way, it was more than I had in years at this point. Dr. Rubin confirmed the diagnosis of RSD. I had some relief from my pain for the first time since the accident and I had an answer. Although the pain was not completely gone, it was only a four on the pain scale versus the usual ten. This lasted for almost three hours and then the pain returned. It hit me so hard that it was like I had to adjust to the pain level of a nine through ten all over again. On my next visit, he told me about how he could do a procedure called pulsed radiofrequency ablation (prfa). It was a similar setup, but the relief could last weeks, months, and even years. I was skeptical, but if I could just have a few more hours of relief again, it would be worth it. Dr. Rubin and Paul, started working out of the same office building were giving me the best treatment I could ask for. One day there may be a cure, or a better treatment but for now, I will take any relief they offer me.

The relief... after the prfa, was not significant. I became sick, stiff-necked, and feverish for days. Every single time and I underwent 36 of them and 37 nerve blocks. I thought that this treatment did not work for me at first. As many treatments, do not work on all RSD patients. Then after a few days I noticed that I did have some relief, my pain was lowered from a 9 level to a 6 level. It lasted up to 23 days, and then the pain returned full force. When I went back to see Dr. Rubin we knew this was a promising treatment option for me. Since then, I have had similar results almost every time. Every four to six weeks I received the prfa and have great success after a few days of bad side effects each time up until December 2008.

At one point, Dr. Rubin wanted to try a full-blown RF procedure instead of the pulsed. We thought that the relief might be greater and went for it. Unfortunately, the few days of horrible side effects turned into three weeks. I went back to him and asked for another procedure after only three weeks. He thought that might be too soon, but it was worth a try. He went back to the prfa and it worked! For some people with RSD this form of treatment only lasts for up to six procedures. With 36 under my belt and still getting relief. Dr. Rubin has agreed to perform the procedure on me as often as I needed. Our hope is that one of these future treatments will be the one that last years for me. Until then, I thank God that He brought me to Dr. Rubin and that Dr. Rubin was informed and knowledgeable in RSD. He helps RSD and chronic pain patients, as well as me, to lead lives that are more enjoyable. With Dr. Rubin, we are treated like people who just happen to have a chronic pain condition. He does not allow me to fall into the trap of my disease becoming me; it is just something in me. Finding a doctor that is willing to help is so important. Do not settle for less! You do not have to settle so don't!

By the time, Dr. Rubin diagnosed me I had dystonia in my right arm, hand and right foot. I was using a wheelchair to get around and life was very limited. I know many people who are afraid to use assistive devices but for me it was freeing to have a way to do something in life. What good was I if I laid in bed every day, crawling to the bathroom and having to have others help me with all aspects of life from cooking, taking a shower and doing anything physical? A wheelchair gave me some freedom.

Willing to do anything to get out of pain, I went into the hospital to have my first rib taken out to make room for my nerves and blood flow. I thought that this would fix all my pain, but I was wrong. The surgeon did a poor job with the surgery and I ended up with spurs growing on my stump of a rib and pain much more severe than I had at the start. After five lung collapses, I went to a new surgeon. He did a body scan in 3-D and saw the problem right away. One spur was hooked into my nerve bundle in my shoulder and the other went directly into my right lung. I had surgery a few days later the rib to remove these spurs.

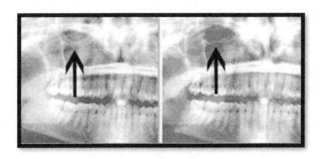

Barby's facial x-ray from the dentist 2004 and 2006.
Note the dystrophy and thinning bone above the top jaw.

Since about a month after the accident, I attended physical therapy, which was excruciating and seemed to make things worse. Finally, in May of 2005, I found my way to a pain clinic here in Arizona. My doctor took the time to listen to my history and look at me. The thought of being examined again was frightening. After an hour with me, he said he thought I had Reflex Sympathetic Dystrophy (RSD) and wanted to run yet another test. He told me he was going to stick a needle into my neck and put a chemical of some sort in my ganglion nerve bundle. If the test worked and the pain was helped even for a short time, it meant that I did have RSD, as all my signs and symptoms had pointed to all this time.

The thing is, I had a doctor, four months earlier, tell me that he was 100 percent sure that I did not have RSD. This same doctor did an electromyography (EMG) on me 6 times, which was awful enough, so the thought of a test that involved a needle was beyond scary. I had found a site on the web and put in my symptoms, even the ones that did not seem to fit with the others. After the site led me to www.chronic painhope.org, I was sure I had the symptoms. Why didn't my original doctors believe me? They saw the symptoms, saw me walk into walls and pass out from the severe pain and more. When my new doctor, Dr. Mark Rubin, suggested that I might have RSD, my first response was, "Dr. Steier was sure I did not." But what test had Dr. Steier done to be so sure? NOT ONE!

After finding so little information out there and having so many doctors, who did not know about RDS, try to treat me, I realized that I am the one who should teach my caretakers. While teaching them, I have learned so much myself that I was inspired to write this book. I have included tools I wish I had in my starting stages of RSD. I want you to have the whole story. In my research, I have found very little literature that tells the whole story; I know how important it is to have the big picture. What information is out there? What is fact and what is fiction? What is old news and what are the newest options for patients?

Chronic or life-threatening illnesses can have a devastating impact on your entire life. I have come to realize that I am the only one responsible for my health. Many doctors who are not connected with a research hospital or university do not have the time to keep up to the minute with the latest information. RSD is just one type of chronic pain. It does not always respond to treatments that other chronic pain conditions would be regularly helped by, though. Even among RSD patients there are differences in response to treatments, as RSD is a fluid disease.

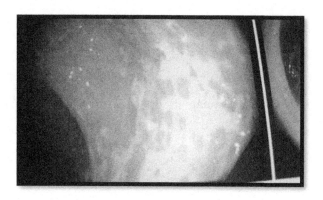

A Picture Showing Barby's Intestinal Ischemia

Sharing this information with you in an easy to understand language has come to be my purpose. If I had a resource like this when I started, I would have spent a lot less time, money and frustration. As I have come to know, RSD does not yet have a cure and only a small number of chronic Pain'ers will ever go into remission. Do not lose hope. There is research going on and the government is taking notice of this debilitating syndrome.

Chronic pain can be a lifelong condition that can have a significant impact not only on the patient but on family and friends as well. The condition affects many aspects of the patient's life in varying degrees. For me, the simple things are the toughest. Daily living activities such as personal grooming, as well as my social and personal life, have all been affected. I lost my professional life to the bad days of chronic pain diseases, also due to not being prepared for a catastrophic injury. I have had to adjust my daily routine because of the inability and difficulty of performing work-related tasks.

I participate in very limited leisure activities as I had to find my tolerance levels and work within them. I used to be very athletic and loved hiking, biking, and dancing. I constantly worked out and trained. Now I have a limited exercise regimen. Because of my pain, falls and blackouts as well as medication side effects, I am no longer able to drive. I need assistance with shopping, cooking, remembering things and traveling. I am in constant need of help, which makes traveling, social activities, personal care and holidays more complicated. I have difficulty sleeping and experience stress in my daily life. All these combined, as well as financial issues and lack of energy, help the cycle of pain continue. Over time, I have found that pre-planning for daily events, activities and trips is not something I should do out of convenience; it is something

I *should do* to be able to function at even a basic capacity. I created a journal, tracked activities and developed plans to accomplish my goals physically.

Financially, I was wiped out. Chronic pain created a financial strain on my family and me. Because of my lack of income and my medical expenses, chronic pain has placed an additional burden on everyone in my life. I am lucky to have qualified for social security disability, while many RSD'ers and other chronic pain sufferers have not. Staying on top of my finances and setting out a plan has helped me reduce stress in this area. Getting advice from a tax accountant or financial planner can also reduce stress levels for patients and their families.

Overall, studies show that quality of life for patients with a RSD is lower than those with other chronic diseases and chronic pain. People suffering with diabetes, migraines and chronic lung disease all score higher in quality of life studies. Despite this, I find that prayer, having a low stress lifestyle, and hope keeps me in a positive place mentally. I have learned not to sweat the small stuff, to let go of troubles from the past and look for ways to better my future. With a good team around you, the same is possible for you.

Living with a chronic pain disease is an invisible disability most of the time. It is harder to get ahead or be understood when you have an invisible disability. Often, people have misconceptions about people with disabilities, and some employers may not consider hiring you if they know about your disability. One of the challenging aspects of dealing with my RSD and other chronic pain diseases is deciding when, or if, I should disclose it to the people I meet. I choose to disclose my condition to anyone who will listen to let them know that chronic pain diseases exist and because of the importance of early detection and proper treatment to chances of remission. The more people I educate, the bigger the chances that someone else who has a chronic pain disease will have it easier. I am strong and am not bothered by the people who believe I might be making it up for attention or other reasons. I know what I live and I want to help others. Not everyone is able to do this. There are some suggestions in later chapters of this book that address when and how to disclose your chronic pain or other invisible disability.

If you are the spouse of a pain patient and you have children, you may worry about the effect of the pain on them. Be sure to include your children. Children often grieve that the new disability is something they caused or something they can cure. My nephew came to visit and I was having a bad day. He asked his mother if he could give me some hot chocolate and cookies to make me feel better. She did not know how to explain to him that this condition was permanent and, although I appreciate the gesture, I am going to always need some assistance and may not always feel good.

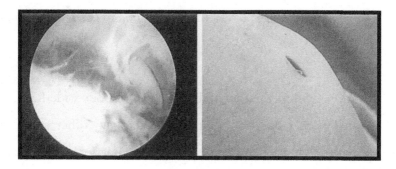

Barby's Shoulder Surgery

Unfortunately, the pain causes our personalities to change and affects the family and friends around us. Most people will never truly understand the physical pain and emotional pain chronic pain patients endure. They will never know how strong you must be to deal with such life changing issues. Finding something to give you purpose can be your saving grace. Taking a job from home, volunteering for an organization or finding someone to mentor can be done if you are upfront from the start and let the people know that you have good days and moments and at times you may have to back out of things. Even now, I need extra time when given a project to accomplish and that can become overwhelming for me. Making sure the person I am working with understands ahead of time helps keep the lines of communication open, set expectations, and allows me to continue to offer something to society.

Along with the extreme physical pain of body wide RSD, and many other pain conditions, it affects many other facets of a patient's life. The extreme changes in your social life, the loss of physical relationships, and the fight against depression are constant struggles.

You can live through it and you can have a greater purpose in life. Life is not over until you die or choose not to LIVE. There are times I feel like I am going to die from this pain, but I don't; I get through it. I have learned to turn to prayer and believe that I deep down want to do my best to live my life as much as I can on my own. If you are unable to get out, you can find others going through similar struggles through the Internet. Learn through trial and error, get involved, and have a greater reason to get out of bed. Concentrate on the great things in your life rather than the pain and negative situation you must deal with. How you look at life will change how you live your life. As we fight and speak out and if there are others like us, we can choose to LIVE. Letting others know they are not alone helps them and can in turn help you. After the accident, I continued with counseling for six months and then have went off and on after I found out that this chronic pain management was going to be permanent in my life.

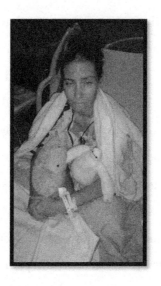

Barby During a Hospital Stay

In September 2007, I could attend an American Association for Pain Management (AAPM) meeting for healthcare workers. At this event, Dr. Schwartzman, a leading specialist of RSD in the United States and internationally, presented the Keynote speech. He spoke about Ketamine infusions becoming the most common future treatment for all RSD patients. After his keynote speech, I had the opportunity to speak to him privately for over 30 minutes. We spoke about my story, what I was doing for treatments, and if there was a possibility that it could be affecting me in a negative way over the long term. His opinion was that it was not going to have a negative impact and, if it was working, to keep going until I could get in to see him. I know RSD patients who have been treated by him with Lidocaine and Ketamine infusions who had great success. I asked him if he would be willing to have me as a patient. He told me to call his office and make an appointment. So, I did.

The earliest date I could get was almost two years later. I think Dr. Rubin and his staff here in Phoenix, Arizona is incredible, but they do not offer the Ketamine infusion. Ketamine infusion is a non-invasive procedure that has shown great potential and promise for remission with RSD patients. I cannot pass up this opportunity but am very fortunate that I have a place to turn to if the Ketamine treatment does not work. My doctors here in AZ are all pulling for me. Although I will not get my life back, I am proud of my accomplishments and am happy that I got to live out my dreams before chronic pain. I now look forward to the day that I can live a more normal life: to work, drive and socialize again. I must constantly be careful of new injuries, but I will physically be able to progress in life.

In 2002, I was in a minor car accident and diagnosed with whiplash. After months of getting worse and noticing new symptoms, I was diagnosed with a shoulder injury and depression, having many doctors tell me it was all in my head. Many of the tests performed did not show any problems. Even so, my symptoms were still bad and becoming detrimental. I went to see over 35 doctors. One doctor performed a vascular study on me and found a lack of blood flow to my right arm, neck and face. He insisted that I needed surgery right away.

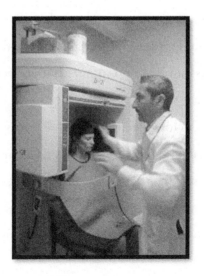

Barby Getting a CAT Scan with Dr. Demerjian, D.D.S.

The importance of a prompt diagnosis is that early treatment is equivalent to higher chances of remission or a lowering of symptoms, in comparison to a later treatment. In my experience, many doctors either have never heard of or do not know all they should about RSD. Many will run tests such as MRI, MRA, X-Rays, EMG, heart tests, vision, hearing, and so on. I even had a dentist tell me I have TMJ based on the pain in the right side of my face. As discussed previously, the likelihood of any other underlying medical condition that could cause the level of pain or dysfunction being experienced by the patient must be ruled out. These issues lead to delayed diagnosis and fewer chances to correct or put the RSD into remission. Earlier diagnosis will lead to better treatment options, preserve mobility, prevent emotional issues and help deal with this nasty syndrome.

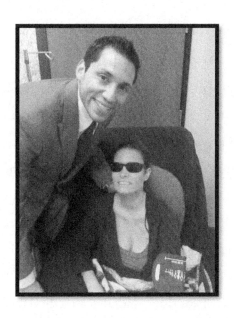

Barby And Dr. Cornidez After an Infusion Procedure

Until a few years ago, there was no way to test for or confirm RSD. Far too often, patients are not believed because there is no way objectively to measure pain. New information has become available and hopes for a possible single test are on the horizon. Currently, there is no single test for RSD available in the United States. Every patient must be diagnosed by the physician based on the patient's history, physical examination, tests to rule out other causes and more tests for changes in pathology. More research needs to be done, but these guidelines are a step in the right direction.

Professionals on a regularly basis are now using a few tests and procedures that are appropriate for diagnosing RSD. These tests include: thermogram, ganglion nerve block, small nerve biopsy, and a patient's clinical history (signs and symptoms). In addition, X-rays can show thinning of bones (osteoporosis), and Functional MRI Nuclear Bone Scans can show characteristic uptake patterns. These testes help diagnose RSD. Unfortunately, there is no specific blood test or other single diagnostic test that can confirm a RSD diagnosis available in the United States, yet.

The test used to find out if I had RSD was the sympathetic nerve block (SNB). There are some advantages to this procedure as a test for RSD. If you are positive for RSD in your upper extremity, after administering the SNB, you will have almost instant relief. However, the drawbacks are that the relief does not last, and you may still be positive for RSD, even if no relief was apparent.

BUILDING A NEW LIFE

I had moved to Arizona for medical care amid divorcing my husband, trying to make it work and realizing once we moved to Arizona together that it was just not going to work. We moved from Washington State to Arizona into my mother in law and step-father in laws house. We were there about a month and then got our own apartment down the road while we were looking for a house. I was in so much pain physically and trying to rebuild my relationship and new life and choreograph the new materials for that summer camp season that was coming up. We met a few of our neighbors and made friends with them.

We then found a house about 30 miles from where we were living and moved in. The first few weeks went well. I was still going to physical therapy, and passing out a lot. The doctors said I was fine to drive though. One day on the way to physical therapy I passed out on the highway when trying to change lanes. The doctors then said I was unable to drive any longer. I started paying for taxi's and friends to help drive me to and from physical therapy. My husband and I decided that we were no longer going to remain married and that it was best to split. At first I left. I stayed on the couch at a few friend's house and my ex stayed at the home we bought. When he realized that I was having to have my rib removed and that my father, mother, and siblings were coming out to help me he moved from the house and I moved back in.

My current husband Ken was one of the first people we met here in Arizona. I ended up paying him and a few others to drive me to appointments. During this time, I made it clear to him and everyone around, I didn't want a relationship, how much I had lost of myself and my life. I had a long way to go to work myself back to where I was physically and emotionally. Over the next year, we became good friends and he became my roommate. Eventually in the summer of 2004 we went on our first date. We went to get ice cream after physical therapy. I think it strengthened our relationship that we were friends first. He really got to see the physical condition I was in, who I was when I didn't have energy to put up a false reality like I did with my first husband. Life was too short and we both knew it. In May 2005 after one year of dating, he proposed to me. We had decided that we would get married once I was physically doing better. His employer at the time allowed domestic partners to be on health insurance and I was covered under his policy and through Medicare and social security disability.

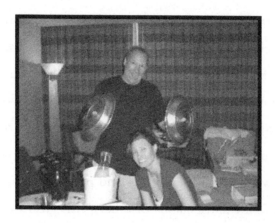

Barby and Ken the Morning After Our Wedding

In November 2007, his company changed their policy and although I was not yet where I wanted to be physically, we knew that Dr. Schwartzman was going to be helping me and soon things would change. We planned our wedding in Vegas and a week later we were married. It was so simple and stress free. Exactly what we both needed. Here we are celebrating our 10-year wedding anniversary this year and are doing better than ever. I learned so much in my first marriage and in living with complicated medical conditions. Ken has been a great life partner for me. A true angel every step of the way.

In 2006, Ken and my family started the nonprofit charity International Pain Foundation (formerly known as Power of Pain Foundation) in my honor to help stop what happened to me from happening to others. We have grown into an international voice for people in pain and are so happy to be working together to make a difference in the lives of millions around the world. With the International Pain Foundation, we know we are changing lives and pain care policy that affects our future and millions of others. It is great to be doing this together and with the support of thousands of others now.

BELIEVING

One of my greatest frustrations has been the lack of an explanation for the symptoms of RSD and why it starts in the first place. Recently, a study by co-authors Julia Rissmiller; Lisa Gelman; Li Zheng, MD, Ph.D; Yuchiao Chang, Ph.D; and Ralph Gott, all from the Massachusetts General Hospital, has identified a cause of RSD. This takes RSD out of the realm of "it is all in your head" or an emotional disturbance. As I quickly found out, many people are skeptical and some physicians are reluctant to treat you. Doctors sometimes see RSD patients as complainers or malingerers. The willingness to show any sensitivity is lacking from these doctors and caretakers.

If you find yourself with a doctor like this, I suggest you get a new doctor, but do not give up on finding some relief for your RSD. For our families, doctors, and our own peace of mind, we need to focus on why the same injuries cause long-term problems in some patients but not in others. This may help lead to a better way of diagnosing RSD, create new treatments and help support groups and family members comprehend the changes that are occurring.

In September '07, Dr Robert Schwartzman addressed the members of the American Association of Pain Management as the keynote speaker. He started by saying, "I finally have something to report."[4] He reported his findings and documentation on how RSD works at a biochemical level, how it affects us inside our brains (because of chronic pain disease development, not the other way around), and that because now that we know how it develops, we can find a cure. There is hope for us. RSD is fully reversible and, per Dr. Schwartzman, "We just have to find the way to reverse it." Effects of RSD can be reversed, plus patients have better chances of recovery and remission.

The symptoms of chronic pain diseases vary from patient to patient and even those with the same conditions. If the patient has not been properly diagnosed yet, these symptoms can cause extreme duress and confusion to all involved. It is

---

[4] Dr. Robert Schwartzman, Keynote speaker for the American Association of Pain Management conference in Las Vegas, Sept 2007

important to get proper diagnosis for what you are living with as the treatment options are so varied with each condition.

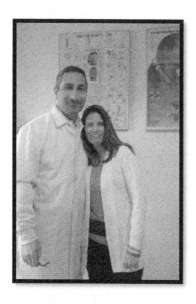

Barby and Dr. Demerjian, D.D.S.

When it comes to reflex sympathetic dystrophy, there are four main categories for our symptoms. The categories are constant chronic burning pain, emotional disturbances, inflammation, and spasms in blood vessels and muscles of the extremities. You should have at least one symptom in three of the four categories to be diagnosed with RSD.

These categories have their own symptoms associated with them. Symptoms include pain, swelling, sweating, spasms, emotional disturbances, short-term memory problems, sleep disorder, and other medical issues. Some effects of RSD can be reversed to give patients a better chance at remission. As the RSD takes over the body, we tend to have a personality change. We grow irritable, anxious; our suffering is evident in our actions and changing expressions. Sleeping becomes a problem. For many of us, being in one position for too long increases the pain levels. We are often jarred from sleep by severe, sharp and burning pain.

I also experience a feeling of electric shock, which can come at any time. I have dropped many plates, drinks and anything I was trying to hold onto from these sudden shocks. As I lose sleep, I also have an increase in hypersensitivity. The heightened sensitivity causes simple things such as a breeze, light or a loud noise to increase the pain. These drastic symptoms are usually caused by a minor injury, which is one of the hardest things to comprehend about RSD.

- Pain

- o "Aching, burning, crushing, dull, electric, feeling as if you're on fire, sharp, stabbing, throbbing, tingling" are some ways to describe the pain.
- o The pain can be anywhere around the affected area, not always right on the site of the trauma.
- o The affected area is usually hot or cold to the touch.
- o The pain will be more severe than expected for the type of injury sustained.
- o The affected area has a lowered threshold to pain from external stimuli.
- Extreme sensitivity to touch: something as simple as a slight touch, clothing, sheets, even a breeze across the skin on the affected area can cause extreme pain to the patient
- Sounds and vibrations, especially sharp sudden sounds and deep vibrations, can also increase pain.
- The softest touch can now cause pain instead of pleasure.
- Sweating
  - o An increase usually occurs

- Spasms
  - The spasms can be confined to one area or be rolling in nature; moving up and down the leg, arm, or back.
- Body fatigue
- Coldness in the affected extremity
- Dystonia
- Tremors
  - Muscle cramps
- Swelling
  - It takes various forms: the skin may appear mottled, become easily bruised, or have a shiny, dry, red, and tight look to it.
  - Swelling is not always present.
  - Swelling can spread to involve a larger area and becomes brawny (hard).
  - Muscle and skin tightness
  - Edema - swelling that is usually localized to the affected limb and may have a well demarcated edge.
- Emotional Disturbances

- o Depression
- o Chronic pain causes depression, NOT the other way around
- o Agitation
- o Irritability
- Short-term memory problems
  - o It becomes easy to lose track of things like whether you took your pills or what you were just talking about.
  - o Loss of short-term memory is a part of chronic pain.
  - o Many patients think they are losing their mind as their ability to remember things greatly decreases, but you are NOT losing your mind.
  - o Other signs of problems here would include the inability to think of, um, well, ah, hmm, just the right word.
  - o The patient's ability to concentrate is also lessened while their irritability is increased.
  - o These problems get even worse as the sleep deprivation cycle continues.
- Sleep Disorder/Insomnia

- o Insomnia is often experienced.
- o Disrupted sleep pattern
- o Inability to let the body drift into rapid eye movement (REM) sleep
- o REM sleep allows the body to use its own healing abilities. Without it, the patient's pain cycle continues and becomes more entrenched.
- o As the body cannot heal itself, it becomes harder to achieve REM sleep, which makes the pain worse and so, the cycle continues.

- • Other Possible Symptoms
  - o Limbic system of the brain
  - o Causes many problems that may not be linked to a disease related to chronic pain at first
  - o Bone Changes
  - o Softening of the bones, Osteoarthritis, Osteoporosis, joint stiffness/ tenderness
  - o Thinning and weakness of your bones become more evident
  - o At risk for more fractures
  - o Nails/Hair on affected extremities, they may grow at a faster/slower rate or become

grooved and brittle
- Hair may become coarse and may be followed by hair loss
- Color/Skin Changes
  - Skin may turn shiny, red, dry and tightened
  - Skin may atrophy
- Balance/Coordination
- Difficulty in beginning or general movement of the injured part
- Dizziness
- General Weakness/ Movement Disorders
- Horner's syndrome
- Increased body fatigue, fever, rashes, sores
- Increased reflex reactions
- Joint stiffness resulting in limited range of motion
- Permanent damage to muscles and joints
- Tinnitus
- Visual disturbances such as blurriness, dry eyes, and others

OFF I GO

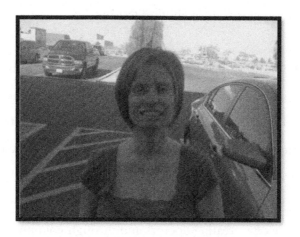

Barby on Her Way to a Doctor's Appointment

A lot of people think remission means: done, I get my life back now. Most people do not realize that remission is a new experience all to itself.

Whether you have been in remission or are still dreaming of it, know that it will be a new chapter in life, and expecting the same life you always knew before your condition set in may not be so realistic. This does not mean it will not be fulfilling, positive, hopeful and a great experience. Chronic conditions such as the neurological condition I have, Reflex Sympathetic Dystrophy, are lifelong changers. The hope and success of remission is still yet another journey.

The healthcare system is not what we are led to believe as we grow up. Doctors are not miracle workers in themselves. They are human just as we all are. We call doctors who treat patients practicing physicians for a reason. People look up to their doctors and put total faith in them. I know I did in the beginning. I have learned through my experience with so many of my own treating doctors and through volunteering with the Power of Pain Foundation that I am responsible for myself, just as you are for yourself. I also learned that doctors study a particular field of medicine. Just because they are neurologists does not mean they can treat both multiple sclerosis and RSD. Each doctor gets a small variety of a medical field and then finds a part of a specialty that they love and work on with great ease.

Unfortunately, so many other patients experience my story. I now want to share my knowledge to lower this number and help those going through the health system at any level. I had to learn the hard way and now want to pass on my knowledge to give hope and answers to patients so they do not have to go through the same. By speaking out about my journey, I am not spewing complaints. I am presenting how I have overcome the challenges presented to me through different experiences.

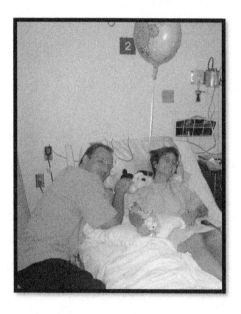

Ken and Barby During a Hospital Stay

What is neuroinflammation and why does it cause such severe burning pain even when there seems to be no injury? Let me explain as simply as I can. Say you sprain your ankle. Your ankle then hurts, swells, discolors, and the pain limits use. The swelling occurs because of "healing" chemicals that move into the affected area and work to heal any damage. In a typical person, this process is successful. This process starts when a healing chemicals triggers another set of chemicals to take the healing chemical away, thus the swelling and discoloration go away. With Reflex Sympathetic Dystrophy, and many other nerve pain related conditions, the second set of chemicals is not activated.

Without that healing process functioning correctly, the prolonged neuroinflammation becomes chronic and activates what we know as glial in your spine and brain. Many specialists in Reflex Sympathetic Dystrophy have said that there is a window of six to nine months to correct this healing process. Others say it is shorter or longer. Nonetheless, this poor healing process "changes your spine and brain" and essentially turns on your pain signals and activates your glia. This often-permanent activation is Reflex Sympathetic Dystrophy.

Glial are small nerve cells that fire off about every two minutes looking for any threats to the body. This is part of your fight or flight system. Glial cells are sometimes called neuroglia or simply glia. They are non-neuronal cells that maintain homeostasis, form myelin, and provide support and protection for the brain's neurons. Glia is a Greek word meaning glue. In the human brain, there is roughly one glia for every neuron with a ratio of about two neurons for every three glia in the cerebral gray matter.[5]

The four main functions of glial cells are to surround neurons and hold them in place, supply nutrients and oxygen to neurons, insulate one neuron from another, to destroy pathogens and remove dead neurons. They also modulate neurotransmission.[6] Therefore, glia is a lot more than just the "glue" of the nervous system. Another well-known item, opioids, also activates glia. I will go into why this is important in an upcoming chapter.

---

[5] Azevedo FA, Carvalho LR, Grinberg LT, Farfel JM, Ferretti RE, Leite RE, Jacob Filho W, Lent R, Herculano-Houzel S. (2009). Equal numbers of neuronal and nonneuronal cells make the human brain an isometrically scaled-up primate brain. J Comp Neurol. 513(5):532-41

[6] FEBS J. 2008 Jul;275(14):3514-26.d- Amino acids in the brain: d-serine in neurotransmission and neurodegeneration. Wolosker H, Dumin E, Balan L, Foltyn VN.

One of the theories I have researched is 'priming of the nervous system'. I can best explain it how Dr. Linda Watkins explained it at a pain conference last year. Let's say that someone slaps you unexpectedly. Your body reacts with a fight or flight response. Then down the road a few months, maybe a year, someone slaps you. Now your fight or flight response is on guard for the situation. It wants to be ready to protect you if any new situation occurs where you may be slapped again. The 'slap' is any trauma. The first can be a torn ligament or broken bone or even a paper cut. The second can be just as big as or smaller than the first incident. The first incident causes the priming. The second confirms the risk, even if there is not one; the body's system is 'on' just in case. Now this is only one theory and it is relatively new, but it makes a lot of sense to me.

I was speaking with a friend who is a research doctor. He explaining to me about a study out of Liverpool that shows Reflex Sympathetic Dystrophy is an neuro-autoimmune disease. A Reflex Sympathetic Dystrophy patient in Canada, who was recently sick, further evidenced this. The doctor put her on an antibiotic and her RSD symptoms disappeared. Once she was well, they took her off the antibiotic and the RSD symptoms returned. Her doctor put her back on the medication and the symptoms disappeared again. This gave the researchers something to base their studies on. If a person has the antigens in their body they have RSD. This test is similar to the one already available for fibromyalgia, only testing for the RSD antigens. They are closer than ever before to an antidote or antibiotic that will target these antigens specifically. This is big news. It is great in the progress of finding a cure. But we are not there yet. It will be many more years until this is the case. I do have hope that this will be life changing for millions of us with RSD.

How is RSD different from other autoimmune conditions? One difference is that the RSD can be in you lying dormant for your whole life and may never affect you negatively. Something your body perceives as a trauma triggers the attack. I can see it also having a negative effect on court cases. RSD is hard enough to explain to a jury now. When the defense throws in that it is autoimmune, I can see a jury becoming confused on what to believe. People would not normally sue if they caught lime disease from a tick bite. This process is easier to explain to the court case participants in states with the 'egg shell law'. Imagine an egg with cracks in it. The egg is still whole, but has some issues. Once something breaks the shell, you cannot put the egg back exactly the way it was prior to the trauma. The egg breaking is the trauma that changes the egg forever, just as an accident or injury is the trauma that changes us forever.

A more positive thought is how this can affect the military. Soldiers are developing Reflex Sympathetic Dystrophy at high rates. If they were able to do this blood test at the time of entry into the armed forces they could screen out potential cases of Reflex Sympathetic Dystrophy development, at least from military injuries for these people. If you knew that you had a propensity for Reflex Sympathetic Dystrophy development, you could live your life a little differently, lowering the chances of a trauma that may change your life.

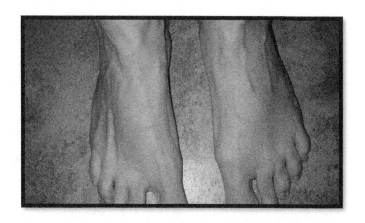

Barby's Feet Showing Atrophy Due To RSD

Here is my time, my chance, my everything, to possibly reverse what I have been living with since 2002. This is my time to go from wheels to heels. My excitement is great, along with the rest of my family. My regular treating doctors are not so optimistic, but are not discouraging either. I believe deep down that Ketamine infusions will put me into remission. I have hope that other doctors around the country will begin to do the protocol that Dr. Schwartzman is using, and more RSD'ers will reap the benefits sooner. I know my doctor here in Arizona, Dr. Steven Siwek, is working with a local hospital to provide it, and in the meantime, he is providing me IV-

Ketamine boosters as an outpatient, using Dr. Schwartzman's protocol.

February 2009, the anticipation of this journey is coming to a head. One of the leading RSD specialists in the United States is Dr. Robert Schwartzman. I have heard others say that their wait was up to five years to get in to see him. I have been on Dr. Schwartzman's waiting list for IV-Ketamine infusions since 2007. Here I am, two years later, leaving in a few days for my appointment in Pennsylvania. This procedure can be life changing. I have so many friends that the infusion therapy helped, so my hopes are high and my belief is soaring.

Since 2002, when my auto accident occurred, all I want is to get better and get my life back. All that has happened up to this point is that I have become weaker physically, and my entire body is now affected, including my heart, intestines, immune system and more. The neurological condition, Reflex Sympathetic Dystrophy, is a stress producer on your body as well as your mind. It affects all aspects of life just as all chronic illnesses do. The strain of financial stress, marital pressure, family expectations and loss of social life can be devastating if you do not keep your life challenges in perspective.

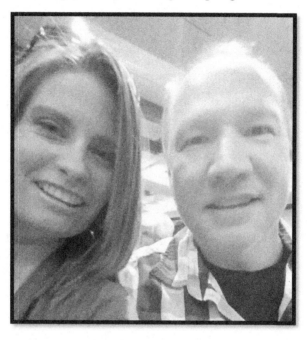

Ken and Barby on a Good Day

March 2009, I was suppose be in Pennsylvania in February to see Dr. Schwartzman, but my appointment was moved to March 30, 2009. I fly out later this month and will be out on the east coast for about a month. I am saddened by the delay but know that there is good reason. Others still have years to wait, so I cannot complain.

Coincidently, at the time my appointment was moved back a month, Dr. Schwartzman was on national news because of complications that occurred with one of his patients in Germany who was undergoing the IV-Ketamine coma treatment. From news reports, I found the problem was not with the IV-Ketamine, but rather the female patient had the MRSA infection, and she had it even before leaving the United States. The virus caused complications and additional bills that her family was not expecting to incur. I still feel fully confident in the process and am moving ahead. I understand that people are upset with the process and don't understand why it costs so much, or why many doctors are not choosing to perform this treatment that the FDA approved and proven to be effective in many Neuropathy pain patients. I know not all patients respond to Ketamine treatments, but this is a noninvasive procedure that has three levels of treatment depending on what state you are in with all of the neurological symptoms and burning pain.

Dr. Schwartzman saw me on March 30. He also had seven other internists with him during the exam. I learned a lot. The bad news I received that day was that I am full body Reflex Sympathetic Dystrophy. I am experiencing sympathetically independent pain vs. sympathetically mediated pain. It is a lot more difficult to treat SIP and his suggestion is now that I go for Ketamine coma.

As it turns out, I was not going for the infusion. I was going for a consult. I am on a waiting list that could take just months or up to two years. I thought that I could see Dr. Schwartzman, have a few days of testing and then begin outpatient Ketamine treatments. After his consult and neurological test, it was evident that this plan was not going to work and that I needed much more invasive treatment than I ever imagined. So, I headed home to see Ken.

I came home to Arizona and have a lot of thinking to do in preparation for my treatments. I am not sure what I want to do. I have been depressed since the visit with Dr. Schwartzman. I have always been strong mentally while dealing with the challenges of Reflex Sympathetic Dystrophy. This time, I was having great trouble getting over the news I heard. It took me over a month to come out of the depression. In the meantime, I am on the waiting list for the coma and inpatient ICU infusions. Whichever comes up first is what I will do.

It is weird to go through this process. I feel like I am on a waiting list for a kidney that is going to save my life. I am just waiting for a bed in an ICU unit, in one of the only hospital in the United States doing this procedure, or a bed in a Mexican hospital to have the coma treatment. I found out that Medicare covers 80% of the infusions done in the United States but I must raise $40,000 for the coma procedure. At this point, I am leaning towards the infusion procedure and will then do the coma if maximum results are not achieved. Dr. Schwartzman thought that the coma could prove to give me 100% effectiveness vs. the infusion that is estimated at 80% effectiveness at best. I have a thick packet to read through over the next few weeks. I will give updates of what I am learning. My wait for the coma may be up to two years and I return to Pennsylvania for more testing in mid-May. This time, my husband gets to go with me.

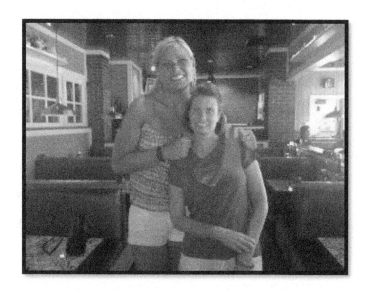

Barby and a friend Amanda

NOT WHAT I EXPECTED

So, what happened during the appointment? When I arrived at Dr. Schwartzman's office, I was excited. I was with my sister and her husband who live in Virginia. Ken did not come with me this time because he had to work. When I start the infusion, I will be isolated for the week anyway and he would be sitting here bored. My family only lives a few hours away from Pennsylvania so it was an easy drive after a long flight across the country. I am hurting all over and many of my symptoms are flaring. I have many types of pain going on right now: burning, stabbing, electric, shooting, deep, surface, bone. I am dizzy from it. Feeling nauseated does not help either.

My name is finally called and my sister and I go the examining room. The nurse is very nice and asks all the right questions. We told her that we'd like to document everything and asked if it would it be okay if we taped the exam. She did not see a problem with it but said the doctor would have the final say. I had also brought the doctor a copy of my book, *RSD in Me!* I was very excited to give it to him, since I spoke about him in one of the chapters. We had previously met in Las Vegas during a conference for the American Academy of Pain Management.

When he had walked into the room to see me, his first words were, "Now she has Reflex Sympathetic Dystrophy. Anyone should be able to see it at first glance." Not all of the doctors who had previously treated me could recognize the symptoms that I had Reflex Sympathetic Dystrophy, and their knowledge was limited. He then began pointing out all of the symptoms, or as I saw it, the flaws I had from the Reflex Sympathetic Dystrophy. He knew things before I even said anything. I did not know to say anything, because I did not know all that was involved.

They had me put on a gown when I came into the room. The doctors saw the blanching from head to toe. From my face to my feet, I had discoloration. I never paid that much attention to how bad it had gotten over the years; maybe because it happened over time. I took pictures of it over the last few years, but did not know it meant that Reflex Sympathetic Dystrophy was in that area. The more severe burning pain was on the right side of my body. Although I had all the other types of pain on the left side, the symptoms of atrophy and coordination were not as bad. I greeted and passed him my book. He recognized me from the conference in Vegas and he seemed to recall my case. I was worse now than I was two years ago. He thanked me for my book and then I introduced him to my sister and he continued with the exam.

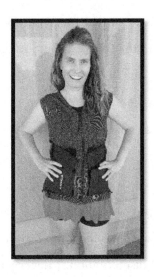

Barby Wearing Her Alignmed Posture Vest

When he began to do the neurological testing on both sides, I felt the pain. The right side was worse, but the left side was affected. He discussed me being diagnosed incorrectly by my other doctors with Thoracic Outlet Syndrome near the beginning of this process and having my rib removed twice with my other doctors. He guessed correctly that I had been diagnosed with TMJ because of the facial pain and that I was having issues with my thyroid. He remarked about the sweating, swelling in areas, asked about my low-grade fevers, Horner's syndrome and more. He noted the atrophy in my hands, arms, legs, feet, face, back and the dystonia in my hands and feet. By discussed, I mean he discussed it with the other doctors. He hardly spoke to me.

Next, he had me do neurological tests. An easy one that you can do right now only involves your hand. Take the tip of your pointer finger and tap it to the tip of your thumb as many times and as fast as you can. I thought that I did it very well, especially on the left hand. He explained how I did it, awkward and slow, was another symptom. I did not understand, so he showed me. He could tap his fingers so fast that it looked like I was going in slow motion. Since then, I ask others to do the same thing. I am amazed that I cannot go that fast no matter how hard I try.

He watched me smile, had me stick my tongue out and then asked me if I have trouble swallowing and does my voice go in and out sometimes. I said, "Yes, how did you know?" He said that the Reflex Sympathetic Dystrophy was affecting my throat and intestines.

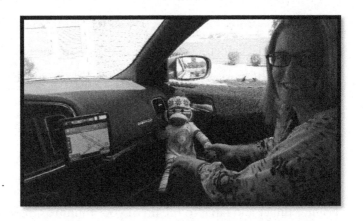

Barby Going on a Road Trip with Her Friend Jose'

I had been diagnosed with gastrointestinal ischemia a few years back. The hospitalist that performed the tests said there is a section of my intestines that is getting little to no blood. I did not understand just how it was related to the Reflex Sympathetic Dystrophy until this visit when I learned that with Reflex Sympathetic Dystrophy you have vascular constriction.

Vascular constriction makes it difficult to get an IV line inserted or even do blood tests. I never realized that the constriction could also affect organs. I thought I was just eating too quickly or being lazy when I choked on food. I did not know why my voice changed or why I would lose it sometimes. The Reflex Sympathetic Dystrophy affected even my nails and hair growth. He was spot on with everything. He added that whiplash or brachia plexus injuries are a leading cause of upper extremity Reflex Sympathetic Dystrophy. With all of my additional traumas and surgeries, the Reflex Sympathetic Dystrophy had spread.

My sister was videotaping and he saw her shaking her head, as he would name off symptoms and issues I had been going through. He stopped, turned to her and asked, "Why are you shaking your head?" She replied, "Everything you are saying is correct. Barby has all of those symptoms." His reply to that was, "You don't know anything. If I gave you a test right now you would not pass it." It was very cold of him, but I can understand where it was coming from. He has worked with Reflex Sympathetic Dystrophy patients, thousands of them, over the last forty years. She is just a sister of a patient with

Reflex Sympathetic Dystrophy. He had seven other doctors in the room that he was trying to teach and more patients to attend to after me.

Dr. Schwartzman made a big deal about this: opioids! He asked if I was taking any. I said Ultram when needed and, rarely, morphine. He told me that if I wanted to do the Ketamine treatments and have it work, I needed to get off all opioids, even Ultram. He also told me to stop radio frequency ablations. When I come back to undergo the IV-Ketamine, they want me in the rawest form, so the system would reboot better. Through his research and working with so many patients, he apparently realized that patients who are on opioids do not have the same results as people who stop them. Since then, I have learned that opioids also set off glia. Therefore, if you are taking opioids and have Reflex Sympathetic Dystrophy you are causing yourself more problems physically, although, you may not care because they also help you mentally escape the pain you are feeling. Dull it, so to say. In addition, he needs you off the opioids because the glia has a Ketamine receptor. In non-technical language, the Ketamine turns off the fight or flight response. If you take a narcotic, you are just turning it back on.

Now, I was ready to hear, "We will do testing over the next few days and then start Ketamine next week." Instead, I got something I never thought I was going to hear.

Sometime near the end of the exam, Dr. Schwartzman was talking to the student doctors about me. He said, "The only thing that will help this patient 100% is the coma treatment." I was in shock. I thought I was going to be getting an outpatient infusion therapy for ten days and then start boosters. I began to tear up. I kept telling myself not to cry. It is never good to cry at the medical doctor's office. I wanted to be taken seriously and be strong. As soon as they left the room, tears flowed down my face. The nurse said she would be right back with all of the instructions and scripts that he was giving me. When she came back into the exam room, she informed us that Dr. Schwartzman was not comfortable with the videotaping and that we needed to erase it. I would have had my sister taking notes if we knew that; we thought we were going to have a videotape of it and there would be no need to take notes. Once we got into the car, my sister told me that she had not erased it. So, we have it for private use and reference, but I cannot make it public.

I did not have any idea of the issues that were involved with Reflex Sympathetic Dystrophy and that I had many of the symptoms. I am now thinking these are going to be some long two years.

I set my sights on preparing. I undergo testing on my heart, lungs, kidneys, liver, x-rays, quantitative sensory testing, and psychological testing. Some of the testing I can do in Arizona. A few of the tests need to be completed with Dr. Schwartzman's specialist.

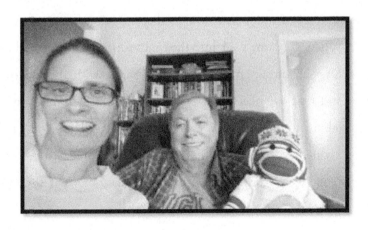

Barby, Her Dad and Jose'

They have to be sure I am physically and mentally ready for the Ketamine treatments. There can be issues so they rule out people who have problems in any of these areas. I do not see myself having trouble in any of the areas, but we will soon find out. I have my dates set for returning to Pennsylvania in May 2009 and have begun my testing that can be done here in Arizona.

Sunday, I rested in Philadelphia at the hotel with my husband to recover from the traveling. Monday morning I reported to Dr. Schwartzman's office and met with two neuropsychology doctors. During the first hour and a half, I was asked questions about my medical history, how I feel about my situation and then some cognitive testing. It all went great. Then, I spent time with the neuropsychiatrist discussing the results and the upcoming Ketamine procedure. Ken could come in for this part. I then went in the waiting room for another hour and a half. I completed a personality test that was multiple-choice. By this time, my pain levels were through the roof and I was on the verge of vomiting, so Ken did all the writing for me. He is the greatest.

Ken ran and got us lunch from the Quizno's across the street from the hospital and doctor's office as soon as we were done with the testing. There were about 300 questions we had to get through. The neuropsychiatrist went over my answers while Ken was gone. He came out to the lobby and let me know that I was cleared for Ketamine on the psychological part and that I was in normal range for what I was going through. As I was finishing my lunch, the next doctor came to get me for autonomic sensory testing (QST-AST).

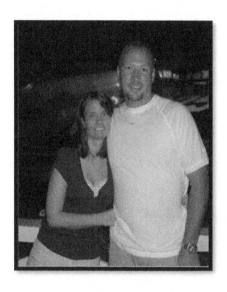

Barby and Ken

The room was like a closet, very small. There was so much equipment in there the doctor had trouble moving it in place at times. I was nervous about how painful these tests would be, but it went fine. First test was a hot/cold test. This test was performed on both of my hands and feet. The device was about 2x1x1 black box, probably made from metal. It is put on two places on each extremity. The test was neat to complete. The doctor heated and cooled the box and it could instantly turn back to room temperature. On my right hand, one of the cold times, I could not hold back from yelling from the pain. I started to tear up. He said I was very sensitive to touch and cold which I already knew. This test was used instead of a nerve biopsy. The doctor said it was more accurate and told them more information than the biopsy would have.

Then, we did a laser picture, it is like a thermogram, but it is more accurate from what I understood. I asked for copies of the picture and it will be a few weeks until I can get it. This laser machine drew out line by line a picture of my thermal image. It was so apparent where the Reflex Sympathetic Dystrophy was from this image. I have been to the Smithsonian Institute in Washington DC where they have a thermogram. You could see the difference with me on that screen but it was not all over as this one was. Still, I drew a crowd at the museum because no one else's scan looked like mine. That scanner was nowhere as sensitive as the one currently being used in Dr. Schwartzman's office. Unfortunately, I am guessing that most people who do the laser thermogram testing for Ketamine clearance have results like mine and it would not be a big deal.

After that, we did a temperature test. He used this handheld thermometer and touched each finger and other parts of my palms and feet to take measurements. They were close in measurements, but with body wide Reflex Sympathetic Dystrophy that is reasonably expected. I remember when it was just in my arm and it was two to five degrees colder than the other arm always.

Next was a vibration test. I thought it was going to hurt. All it entailed was a small black box with a sensor the size of a dime sticking up. I put my index finger and then my pinky on the sensor and he would turn it up. As soon as I felt it, I would tell him and he cut it off.

The final test was a coordination test. You can try it. Take a keyboard and put your thumb below the space bar and your index finger on the key. You might have to have someone hold the keyboard for you. Have someone time sixty seconds while you hit the bar as many times as you can. On my left hand, I got just over seventy and my right was around thirty. He said that the average for a healthy person is 150-170. I thought I was doing well until he said that. I asked him to show me what normal would look like and he did the test. I was amazed at how quick he was. Then the testing was over.

The sensory testing doctor said he was done early because I went through the test so fast due to the sensitivity. I went through the test fast because as soon as you feel it, your measurement is done and you move on. Ken and I then rested for the remainder of the day and prepared to fly home at 4 A.M. EST (1 A.M. our time) to Arizona. Overall, the trip was successful. I do have to get one additional cardiac test done here in Arizona before I can be scheduled for the Ketamine. My EKG test I had in Arizona before I left came back with an abnormal finding and I must more testing. I see my pain doctor in two weeks and my first fundraiser is coming up in June. I am full of hope for the future and happy I could have a good life experience in the mist of all the challenges.

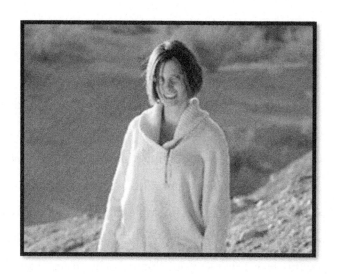

Barby on a Good Day

May 2009, this afternoon I will have my echogram done at the Arizona Heart Institute. Please say prayers that the results come back as normal. I am hoping to be squeezed in for an appointment to have my table tilt test on Tuesday afternoon at a hospital in Phoenix. I also get to see my primary care doctor on Tuesday morning for a checkup.

After this round of exams, I will be ready for the Ketamine procedure. I will let you all know how Monday and Tuesday go. Once again, thanks for the love, support and prayers. Everything you are doing helps!

June 4, 2009, Yesterday was a miserable day. I tried taking Toradol, a non-narcotic pain medication, but within an hour I was vomiting and that continued into the night. I had a spike in my fever, which got up to 102.6 and, of course, had major pain. I did not get in for the table tilt test yet. I am trying again for next Tuesday. Apparently, there are not many places to go for this test. I will let you all know what it was like, hopefully soon.

As far as the echogram, the test went fine. The tech could not give me any results but she did not seem worried about anything she saw. I did not think that this test would hurt as bad as it did. She said the bone is so thick and to see the heart she had to press firm.

Well, when she was pressing between my ribs, it felt like she was trying to separate them! The exam lasted about 15 minutes and she did the pictures in color (showing blood flow), as well in black and white. I could see all four chambers of my heart on the screen. There were also three electrodes attached to me so they could monitor my heart rate, so I could hear my heart beating and it sounded normal to me. I am so ready for all of this to be done.

June 15, 2009, I received my results from my echogram today and they came back normal. I am still waiting for an opening at the hospital for the table tilt exam and hope to hear something by Wednesday. Then, I will be ready for the procedure and all I have to do is raise the remaining funds needed and wait. Yesterday, Ken and I met with a woman from the community who runs a foundation. Their mission is to support people from Arizona in times of need with their medical expenses. Wherever there is need or injustice, they can offer resources regardless of economic status or affiliation. They have offered to assist me in raising the rest of the personal medical funds I need for my Ketamine procedure.

June 25, 2009, I finally got my time and date scheduled for my table tilt exam (cardiac test). It is next Wednesday. I am very excited because this is my last test before Ketamine.

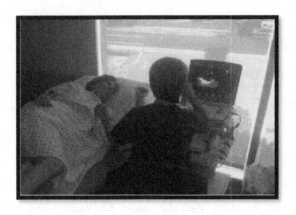

Barby having Heart Echogram

July 18, 2009, I have had a rough few weeks but I did get my table tilt exam and a new EKG. The table tilt exam came back in the low - normal range, however the results of this EKG were the same as the original: abnormal. Despite that, the cardiac doctor approved me for the Ketamine procedure. Now it is a waiting game.

The table tilt exam was different than I expected. They strap you to a table with three straps and then tilt the table up to a 70-degree angle. I was in that position for 40 minutes and I was in sheer pain the whole time. I got a little dizzy and nauseous, but stuck it out so that I could be cleared. My left arm had a blood pressure cuff, IV line and oxygen monitor. My blood pressure was so low that the machine only picked it up every two or three times it tried. Every time the blood pressure check was taken, the IV line would be cut off and blood would come back out the IV tube. By the time that the blood was back in and saline was flowing it was time for another blood pressure check. I do not think I got any IV fluid. Once the test is over, they bring the bed back down so it is parallel with the floor. For me, though, it felt like I was upside down. The feeling lasted about twenty minutes. The cardiac doctor did the repeat EKG, which came back abnormal as I said above. I will see the cardiac doctor in the next few weeks to discuss the exact problem with my heart and what we can do about it, if anything. Reflex Sympathetic Dystrophy does affect your autonomic system, so to me there would be an effect on the heart since it is an 'automatic' organ.

August 18, 2009, I finally got my heart test results and it turns out I have cardiac ischemia. This is when the flow of oxygen-rich blood to the heart muscle is impeded, resulting in inadequate oxygenation of the heart. At the end of this month, I am undergoing a nuclear scan stress test. A nuclear stress test measures blood flow to your heart muscle at rest and during stress. During the test, a radioactive substance is injected into your bloodstream. This substance mixes with your blood and travels to your heart. A special scanner, which detects the radioactive material in your heart, creates images of your heart muscle. After that, I will find out what the cardiologist wants to do.

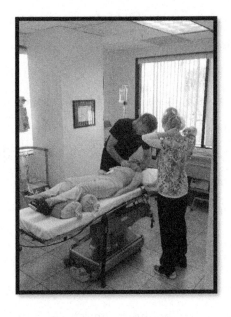

Barby Being Prepped for Her Stem Cell Infusion with Dr. Mark Berman and Nurse

I also got a call from Dr. Schwartzman's nurse letting me know I could be called anytime between now and February 2010. I am excited because I am having some very rough days. Some days I only get through by prayers and hope. Just knowing that there can be an end to this is keeping me going.

In addition to the other testing, I have to get an x-ray of my chest to make sure my lungs are clear. This was an easy test. I was in and out in minutes and everything was normal.

The blood tests have to be done in thirty days or less from when you are heading into the hospital, so those will wait. They do the normal CBC testing, but also check other organ functions and if you have any viruses. I have not been able to have a nurse or doctor draw blood from me since 2007, so it will be interesting to see how they get what they need in these tests. Just getting an IV line in for a radio frequency ablation would be a fiasco. An anesthesiologist would put in the IV line and then my doctor would come in to do the procedure. He would have to manipulate the line in my arm, hand or elbow (where ever they put it) at that moment so I could be given the sedation medicine. Once I would fall asleep I am not sure how much longer it worked, but probably not long, seeing sometimes he had to hold it in place with his hand and it would stop when he let go. I cannot imagine that someone would be assigned to holding my IV line while he performs the procedure.

THE WAITING GAME

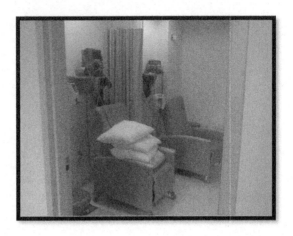

Picture from the Infusion Suite at Drexel Neurological Institute

Now it is time for the wait part of the 'hurry up and wait' life I live. I hurried up and got every test done. Crossed all my dots and dotted all my T's as I like to say. Now it is out of my hands. I am waiting for my bed and just must be patient. In the meantime, I have no relief from the pain except heating pads, a dark, quiet bedroom and my faith that Jesus will bring me through this. Everything will be fine; I just have to make it a few more months. I can do it.

No Meds, No Treatments? What is it like to stop all your pain medications? It can be very scary. I have many friends who this terrifies. I, on the other hand, was glad to get it out of my system. I am thinking clearer. Although I do have to say, Reflex Sympathetic Dystrophy does cause memory problems.

The withdrawal can be the scariest part. I can say that for me it was about two weeks of withdrawal that was really bad, but the rest of the year was still pretty tough due to the increase in pain levels.

My will was to get Ketamine and get my life back. People who are on higher doses may have to go into a rehab program to detoxify. Others will just skip Ketamine because they are afraid to get off the opioids and others will try to do the IV-Ketamine while on opioids. Those of my friends who have done the latter did not have the results I did. They got either temporary relief, as in days or hours, or no relief. Neither were options for me. I was going to follow the protocol exactly, and I did. There is no need to question what is proven to work.

October 21, 2009, Big news! I got the call today from Dr. Schwartzman's office. It is my turn to go for the Ketamine procedure. This will be the five to ten-day inpatient version in Philadelphia, Pennsylvania performed at Drexel University Hospital. I will be in the intensive care unit for that entire time and will be secluded from visitors and outside influences such as my cell phone, internet, and texting. I think it will be harder on my family and friends than it will be on me. The bad news: I still need a significant amount of money to accomplish this. I am working hard to get this done, but I have a feeling of calmness and believe in my heart that it will all come together for me. I surprisingly do not have any anxiety about it at all, the procedure or the money.

I will get a call from Dr. Schwartzman's nurse in a few days to go over last minute procedures.

A few days later, I got a call from Lynn, Dr. Schwartzman's nurse. We were going over all the instructions and she told me to get my blood testing done. I mentioned that I might have to wait until I get to the hospital because they have not been able to draw blood from me for a few years. She told me she was going to speak with Dr. Schwartzman about it. They have other patients who have similar issues. When she called back a few days later, she said Dr. Schwartzman looked at my case and suggested I get a PICC line or a Port-a-catheter. It will make it better for blood draws, as well as keeping a good line for the infusions. I considered it a little and decided on a Port-a-catheter because it could be in for five years, takes a thousand pokes, is under the skin and infection would be less of a risk. Those sounds like great benefits to me. I still have the Port-a-catheter in my chest today (2017) and its doing great 8 years later. The experience of placement of it was not that fun though.

November 10, 2009, Tomorrow I am having a Port-a-catheter put in. This way during the infusion and the following boosters, I will not have to have an IV line or PICC line replaced every few days or months. The Port-a-catheter can stay in for a long period and is often used by cancer patients who are undergoing chemotherapy treatment. Getting an infusion therapy is the same process whether it is a chemo drug, IVIg, Lidocaine, Metamine or, Ketamine. It will take about seven days to heal from this procedure and then the plan is to send me off to Dr. Schwartzman to begin the Ketamine procedure. I will try to get some video of the procedure or at least some photos of the process.

November 11, 2009, before they could take me into surgery, they had to draw blood. I thought that was funny, since I was there to get a Port-a-catheter because they could not get a regular blood draw. The nurse wanted to try, so I let her. After one try, she called over the head nurse. She looked and looked. She just knew she was going to be able to do it. Then they called over a doctor. He looked and looked. Finally, he told them to use an ultra sound machine to locate a vein that would work. They found one: deep inside of my elbow. I am glad I got it right before going into surgery, so when I woke up I would be out of it and would not care about the pain.

The surgeon came into my curtained off area and asked me if I had any questions. I said no. I had had a PICC line in the past a few times and this was similar just on the inside. I did have anxiety about the procedure and was afraid to hear anymore. Now I wish I had asked questions. I should have asked questions. I was not prepared for the major surgery that it is. I did not know that the scars were going to be so big. Not that I am worried about how scars look; I have so many others, but I was not mentally prepared for the recovery. It was a scary, painful and uncomfortable time. In my speeches, I teach other patients to be fully informed for any medical issues they are going through, especially a surgery. I am sorry I did not follow my own advice going into this procedure.

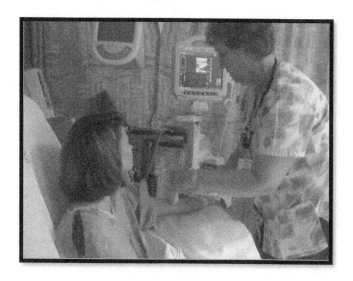

Nurse Had to Use Ultrasound to get a Blood Draw

November 20, 2009, I got my Port-a-catheter placed on November 11. It was much more invasive than I thought it would be. I have a scar on my neck and one on my chest. They still are not healed fully. On November 12, I began running a fever and headed back to hospital to make sure everything was okay. After that visit, it shows no infections were indicated on the test they performed.

Nov. 18th was my birthday! I had to go to the hospital and have the port used to take blood. It was a great experience and it did not hurt. Shocking!

As they tried to get blood on the 12th, the nurse did not do it very well and it was very painful. The access line seemed to be stuck! It took my breath away when she finally yanked it out. The nurse on my birthday was great and I did not feel a thing. I am still having trouble sleeping and getting comfortable and used to having this port in me. I can feel it move especially as the swelling goes down! The nurse said the wound will be tightened back up and I will get used to it. I hope that happens soon.

November 27, 2009, There are so many things I want to do after this Ketamine procedure. I cannot wait to start weight bearing physical therapy. My first goal is to walk to the mailbox and back without help or needing to take a break. My hope is that after the Ketamine procedure, I will be able to continue my fundraising to cover this life-changing procedure and the follow up booster treatments.

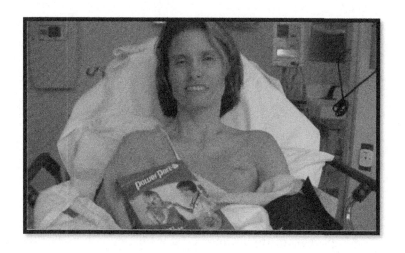

Barby Just Out of Surgery for Portacath

As far as a date to start the Ketamine procedure, I am told it will probably be about January 4, but could be as soon as December 7. The January date will allow me to work on getting the rest of the funding together, as it is a prepay procedure. Earlier in the book, I said that Medicare covers this procedure. Well I happen to be "lucky" in that I have a primary insurance due to my husband working. It is great in all situations except this one. Drexel Hospital said my primary insurance would not cover this procedure. Therefore, my secondary won't either, even though Medicare would cover it if they were primary, I am facing a tough financial situation.

I will be heading out east this Friday, as there is a great chance the Ketamine could start on December 7. This would give me the time to raise or borrow the funds needed; also, just in case a patient cancels. Ken has taken on a second job and will be working weekends and some evenings to help with the financial aspects of this procedure.

My port scars are healing and it is becoming less sensitive. My neck scar is almost undetectable; the one on my chest is healing slower, but getting better. It is quite a weird feeling to have this under my skin and on top of my rib. The port sticks up off me so it is not too discrete, but the benefits are going to be great and I look forward to the ease of it as I go through this process.

December 2, 2009, I leave Friday for Philadelphia. I am so excited!!!!! *\O/* Donations are still needed to offset the ongoing medical expenses that will be incurred as I continue the Ketamine protocol to ensure ongoing remission. For the last seven years, I have had to deal with the daily challenges of a debilitating disease. In basic terms, my nerves (pain) are turned on and stuck that way. I feel like I have been set on fire all the time. I am going to put the fire out!

My doctors have tried all reasonable options. I have undergone one painful, intrusive treatment after another, many of which had side effects almost as bad as the condition itself. My family and friends have had to watch, helplessly as I turned from an energetic, joyful cheerleader and coach to a disabled woman. However, there is one last hope.

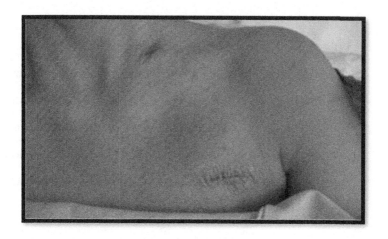

Scars from Portacath Insertion

What is my prognosis without the treatment? Because it took almost three years to diagnose my Reflex Sympathetic Dystrophy condition, it has made the disease extremely difficult to treat. Without this treatment, I will continue to deteriorate. There is always the possibility that if I get the infusion it may not work. I have done everything I can do to have a successful outcome. If, for some reason, it does not work, the pain, along with the progression of the disease and the side effects of the short-term treatments, will continue to take a heavy toll on my body and spirits. As time passes, I will become more and more disabled and need increasing amounts of care and medications. So this just has to work!

Following the procedure, I will receive boosters every few weeks to months, possibly in Pennsylvania. I hope that Dr. Siwek will still do the boosters when we are back in January. Seeing I will be the only patient he is doing this for, at least for the time being, it will be an interesting process. These booster treatments are obviously expensive, but they are vital, and an ongoing part of the infusion therapy.

December 4, 2009, I am about to take off for Pennsylvania. I am excited and hopeful. I have taken out loans for what I did not raise. Some people who promised donations or assistance did not come through, so I ended up taking out medical loans for the rest. While I am in the hospital, Ken will post an update each day. Please keep me in your prayers. So many people ask me about the actual process. I will explain as much as I know.

From Wheels to Heals by Barby Ingle

FAMILY FEELINGS

This chapter is written by Ken Taylor, Barby's husband.

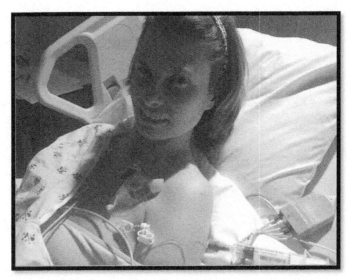

Barby Just Arrived at Drexel University Hospital, Getting Hooked Up and Ready to Start IV-Therapy

It's 12/7/2009 or GO time for Barby! After registration, there is no more contact with the patient. A phone number is given to the family to contact the nurses for updates each day. I spoke to a nurse around 10P.M. It took time to reach the max dose for inpatient medication and my family was told that it takes about six hours to do so. Thus, a follow-up will take place in the morning.

From Wheels to Heals by Barby Ingle   Page | 158

12/8/09- Tuesday morning 10 A.M. - I reached Barby's nurse and was pleasantly informed that everything is going as planned. Barby's nurse, Colleen, told me that Barby is reporting her pain right now to be a zero out of ten, that she is doing very well, and that she is right where she needs to be at this time.

I had to ask again. Colleen repeated, "Barby's pain level is a zero. She is not in pain." I do not know how out of it she is and if she really knows what she is saying at this point. Thank you all for your prayers. Please keep them coming.

12/9/2009- No pain is all gain. Barby had a pain level of zero last night, but this morning it went up while trying to eat a little food. Eating brought on nausea, which brought on the pain, so the nurse gave her some medicine to help both, and she is sleeping just fine now. She is aware of who she is and where she is at, just groggy and a little off, kind of like "she is drunk or drugged up" ...so the good news is that when she is asked about her pain levels, she is aware of how to respond if she is in pain. So, if she says she is in 0-pain level, we should think that she is telling us how she is really feeling.

From Wheels to Heals by Barby Ingle   Page | 159

12/10/2009- Mobility!!! Nurse Chris said, "She is reporting her pain to be at a level three but it will ebb and flow throughout the treatment. As she gains mobility there will come new limits that she will need to learn. The real test comes on day seven when she comes off the Ketamine to see if the pain will stay or go." On a side note, he told me that Barby was watching *So You Think You Can Dance* and was educating him on different dance moves. GO BARBY ;)

2/11/2009 - Jumping for joy. The nurse said Barby is doing very well and is very comfortable where she is. She still has two days left to receive the Ketamine. The treatment protocol is for five full days with an additional day to titrate up, and another day to titrate down. She should be ready to go home on the 14th. I can't wait to see her.

12/12/2009- Great progress! Nurse Colleen said that she is very happy to see Barby's progress and that Barby is on cloud nine. She also said tomorrow is going to be the big test. Then, they will know how much the treatment helped her. So far, all signs are good and they do not see any complications.

12/13/2009- Get ready to go! Colleen said, "Barby remains pain free and ready to go home." She will titrate down tomorrow and be released tomorrow evening sometime. Barby has no pain when stretching her right arm anymore. Her skin color is back to normal. Sweating is gone and she is asking us to bring clothes and shoes that were normally uncomfortable and painful to wear for any length of time. Colleen said, "Barby is ready to go home, experience life on a new level and start living." I will see for myself tomorrow. I can't wait to pick her up. - Ken

12/14/2009- Picking up Barby! Barby's sister, her husband and I are driving to Philadelphia to get Barby out of the hospital. When we called the nurse to find out what time we would be there to get her, the nurse asked if we would like to speak with Barby. Oh, how excited we got. Then Barby got on the phone. She said she did not know what the nurses had been telling us but her pain was not a zero, it was a three. She was very sad and we all got very worried. The rest of the drive we were very confused. Then her sister realized it was the bad weather. It was snowing. That could be the cause of the spike in pain, so we focused on that.

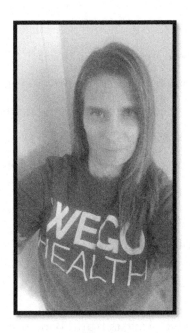

Barby Received The 2016 WEGO Health Lifetime Achievement Award and Helped International Pain Foundation Win The 2016 Best In Team Performance Award

When we got there, Barby looked so good. She was so happy and looked great. Well, she looked good for someone who had been lying in a hospital bed for a week. We noticed her window shades were closed. She did not know what the weather was like all week. When we opened the windows, she was also thinking that the weather was the culprit of her rise in pain.

Barby was still out of it. But we didn't realize how much until later. She had her sister come over so she could tell her a secret. She had saved her Lorna Doone cookies. They are the best in the world she tells us. Her sister said those are not the best. They are only Girl Scout Trefoil cookies and they are crappy. Barby said "Oh" and looked sad for a moment. We brought up another subject and Barby sprung back to life. She forgot the cookies were even spoken about. We videotaped the whole pick up experience to put on YouTube. It was a very great day, happy time and full of joy! As Barby would say, "It is a Shake the Poms moment!" *\o/*

On the way home, we stopped at Outback Steak House to have a celebration dinner. – Ken

WHAT AN EXPERIENCE

12/16/2009- Hey everyone, it works!!! I am finally home. I got home on Sunday night but just coming out of my fog or "k-hole" as many people call it. My burning pain is gone, but I am having another ache. It feels like the deep bone pain, but it is not constant and occurs more when I am overworking. I slept most of the time I was there. They wake you up to eat and try to have you conscious when the doctors come to visit throughout the day, so they can do neurological evaluations to see your progress. Each patient, no matter your size, weight, or whatever, is titrated up to the maximum dose and then held there for five days, so the process takes longer than the five days. I did not know that going in to the hospital.

The first day, they take you up to the maximum dose over many hours. Once there, your five days start. After the five solid days, you come back down over many hours and then have to be observed for more hours before being released. My results were great from the start (at least that is what I remember). I don't remember much after the first night. Some of my accounts are from what was told to me after I was done.

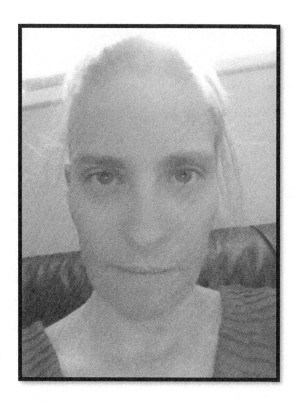

Barby At a Doctor's Appointment In The Waiting Room

Dr. Schwartzman was very excited to see the blanching gone. Yes, gone. My skin is white with no blanching; I need a tan. No sweating, no swelling and best of all, no burning! I did have a catheter in the entire week, except the first and last day. Now

I am having some trouble with urinating and am taking some medication for a urinary tract infection.

I got a call today to set up my first set of boosters on Dec. 28 and 29th. It is a two-day process, which I found out today. So, typically, all of the patients follow the same schedule for boosters. My boosters will be: two weeks after the initial treatment, then again in two, then again at four weeks, and finally three months. Depending on how I am doing, we will do them as needed after that point.

Dr. Schwartzman said, "No PT, still!" He put it like this: They are bad nerves still. He has gotten them to be good, but they are looking for any reason to be bad again. So, I have to be very careful still. That is one of the reasons why it is *Remission* instead of a *Cure*. I also asked him if I could get off my Lamictal medication, which is a seizure medication also prescribed for burning nerve pain. He said no, that my body might perceive it as a trauma. My physical therapy will be learning to live everyday life. Finding my limits and trying activities will be more than enough for me to handle. I will continue to have limitations and much of what I lost with muscle and bone will not come back. I must hold myself back. I thought I was going to be able to do whatever I wanted. This is not the case. However, I am doing more than I have in seven years.

I am still very weak, and my legs are like Jell-O, but I am so glad to go through these life challenges versus the burning pain 24 hours a day, seven days a week. It is worth it, and I suggest all RSD'ers try it.

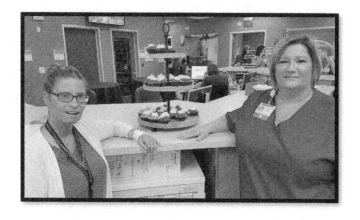

Barby Bringing Treats to the Nurses Who Help Her

I am doing well still. On Thursday, last week, Ken and I went with my little brother, his wife and my newest nephew to a holiday party thrown by his physical therapist. Many of the staff there had read my book and really wanted to meet me in person. With the Ketamine working so well, I was excited to show off. I was shaking hands, proud as could be at my progress. The doctors there were very interested to hear about the process and most had never heard of the IV-Ketamine procedures, so I hope I excited them enough to go and research how easy it is to administer it and how much it can help their patients. We need more doctors doing this Ketamine procedure.

While out, we started noticing that with little to no pain my vision was not doubled, I was walking more upright, as well as the no sweating, blanching, or vomiting. I started to get tired and worn out, and so did my nephew, so we headed back to my sister's house. It was so exciting for me to get out and actually enjoy the experience and meet people. It was also exciting for my family to see me doing so. They say I have a new glow and look of happiness that they have not seen for years. I am feeling very well. I just tire easily.

Dec. 21, 2009- Trip to Dad's. I traveled for eight hours to my dad's house (which is normally a two hour drive at the most) last Friday night. The ride was so long because of the snowstorm that hit the east coast. By the time we got to my dad's house, the pain was an eight to ten level. The burning pain was back. The roads were slow going and there were accidents all over. The stress level was high and on top of that, the car I was in was very bouncy and every "ice rock" we hit reverberated through me. My seatbelt was going over my port (on the left part of my chest), and as the car bounced around, the seatbelt would lock up, causing me more pain.

I tried to sleep during the ride but was able to stay asleep for about an hour. The pain was so intense. I was nauseous from the pain and ready to cry as I thought the pain would never subside again. However, Saturday afternoon, it began to get better. I got to see my older brother and his family (wife and my two nephews) as we had Christmas dinner Saturday evening. I did not try hugging them until the end. Nevertheless, it went great and we did soft hugs before we left. I have only done air hugs up to now since the Reflex Sympathetic Dystrophy went full body and never got to hug them. It was one of my goals to hug my family members if the Ketamine worked. I got to fulfill my goal.

I rested Sunday and watched a couple of movies and the finale of *Survivor*. By then, my pain levels were going down.

It is now Monday morning and I am feeling good. Pain level is about a two in some areas, but most of me is at zero pain level.

We are going to head back to my sister's house in a couple of hours. I pray that it is only a two-hour drive and that the interstate is clear the whole way.

My first Ketamine booster is coming up on December 28th and 29th. Yes, two days. I found that out last week. The boosters are four hours each for two days. I will do this set in Philadelphia at Dr. Schwartzman's office and then hope to have my Arizona pain doctor, Dr. Siwek, take over the administration of the boosters from that point. I will have one due two weeks after I get home (mid-January); one month after that (mid-February), and then after three months (May). At that point, I will be reassessed.

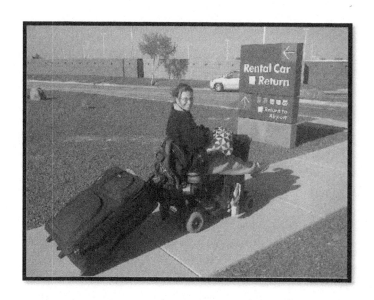

Coming Home After Going into Remission

If I stay in remission, I will not need to do the inpatient version again. However, any trauma can take me backwards and after the car ride to my dad's house I see how little the trauma must be. As Dr. Schwartzman explained, my nerves are still 'bad nerves' that he got to behave, but they still want to be bad so I have to be careful not to give them a reason. If at any point, after the June procedure, I can start the process over if needed. If I come out of remission, and if I have the funding to do so, I would be happy and excited to do it again just to have the relief I have.

From Wheels to Heals by Barby Ingle

Jan 5, 2010 - New Year's Update. Ok, I am back in Arizona and doing well. I got my boosters December 28th-29th, 2009 and I cannot remember much about it.

Here is what I do remember: I arrived at Dr. Schwartzman's infusion suite and signed in. That morning I could not remember if they said to take one or two Ativan, so I took two just to be safe. I remember the nurse called us all back and told us our assigned chairs, and then led us each into a room where our access lines, port line or regular IV line were inserted. That is the last thing I remember until December 31, 2009. Ken says I told him I was out of my body and that I felt like a bunch of blocks.

He adds that when trying to walk I looked like a bunch of blocks, which had to look funny. He said I was doing well until he got me to the hotel room and as he opened the door, I said I was going to throw up and went toward the trashcan. Well, I missed, and of course he had to clean up.

The next day, he told the nurse what had happened and they gave me extra nausea medication so it did not happen again. After the infusion on the second day, Ken drove me back to Virginia.

We spent the next two days at my sister's house and then New Year's Eve with my brother, his wife and my nephew. We headed back to my sister's house at 2A.M. and took a short nap before leaving to the airport at 4A.M.

The flight home was a little bumpy in some places, but it was a straight five-hour flight to Arizona. We had no radio or movie on board, but we both took the opportunity to sleep.

Over the weekend, we went through our mail and were happy to see that we received more donations while back east. We also got a bill from Drexel Hospital for $104,599 as well as doctor, radiology, lab, pharmacy bills for another $10,000. Are you kidding me?

I spoke with the billing department today. We are working on getting some of it negotiated down and taken care of which will be nice, seeing that I had to take out a medical loan for most of the $18,000 I prepaid. It can take up to 45 days to get it all sorted out.

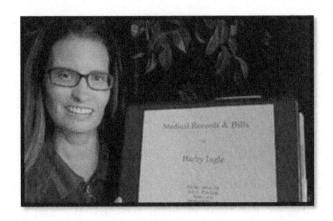

Barby With Her Medical Bill Binder

I am sure that we will be okay! God has brought us this far. I must leave this bill in His hands. I have stayed at 85-100% pain free levels. The burning pain is practically gone. It has tried to sneak in here and there, but then I rest and wake up doing better, or wait for the bad weather to pass. I guess that is what the boosters do. They remind my nervous system to be "good," as well as making me remember Dr. Schwartzman's instructions to do no physical therapy. In the papers sent home with me, it was clear to "avoid injuries!"

We met other patients and their caregivers in Philadelphia at the booster treatments. It was great to exchange information and make some new friends who are going through the same thing. We have already heard from a few of them since arriving back home.

I am waiting to hear from my Arizona pain doctor about doing my next set of boosters here, instead of flying back to Pennsylvania. I do have dates set in Philadelphia, if needed, that I will use in mid-January. I may be making another trip out east real soon. One good thing or bad thing, depending on how you look at it, is that on my trip out to PA, the airline messed up my scooter battery and it will cost more than two hundred and fifty dollars to fix. In place of the battery repair costs, they gave me a free roundtrip ticket so I can fly free on this next trip if needed. Moreover, I am not using my scooter anymore so I have time to get it fixed when we have the money. I don't have to stress about it too, at least, not yet.

Last night, I decided to walk to the mailbox. It is quite far from our house. By the time I got there and put the key in the box, I was already tired, and then I realized that... I had the wrong key. So I had to walk all the way back! Afterward, Ken and I drove to the box with the correct key, as I was hurting too bad to try the walk again. Oh well, I am learning my new limits. My mission is continued remission!

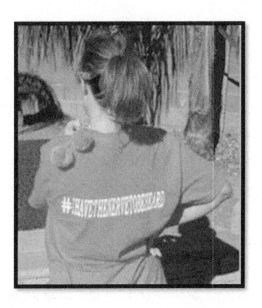

Barby Hast the Nerve to Be Heard – Part of the NERVEmber Project She Created For iPain

January 30, 2010, I am doing well. Thank God. I got word this past week that my third in the set of four mandatory boosters will be on February 18 and 19th. This past Tuesday, I also went to see Dr. Hummel, my primary care doctor, who I spoke about in my first book. He was so shocked at how I was doing. I do not think he thought it was going to work. However, he was very happy for me! I did have blanching that day, but I do not know why. I also had a slight fever.

The highest pain I have had since coming back to Arizona is a level four. That is nothing to complain about. I have not thrown up from pain since before the inpatient procedure in December. My dystonia was better. I had a glow of life that he had never seen and he was just shocked at how I was doing. He opened the exam room door and called the nurses and office staff. "Come look at Barby; I can't believe how she is doing," he said. They came in and were shocked as well. He and his staff never knew me before Reflex Sympathetic Dystrophy. They were now looking at the "after Ketamine Barby" and were so happy for me. I am a new person. Not the same person I was eight years ago, but who is the same person they were eight years ago. Dr. Hummel said he doesn't need to see me unless I have any issues that come up. No more regular doctor visits. Happy day! I wanted to go back to what I was before this all happened to me. I am going to work hard to do all of the things I am not able to do. However, I am finding that I have limits that I did not expect to face.

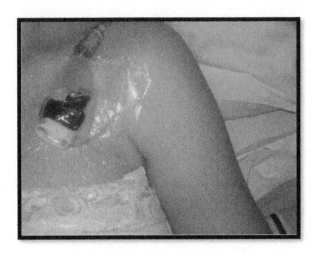

Getting Hooked Up for First Booster In Arizona

At the same time, I am doing some laundry and dishes. I have tried sweeping and that is still painful and difficult for me to do, so I stopped. I am putting dishes away, hanging clothes, and I even did some ironing. I am awake more and have energy that I didn't know I had, although there has been limits to that as well. Ken has to adjust to what I am now able to do; it has to be weird for him. He has never seen me do most of this before going through the IV-Ketamine because I simply was not able to do so.

January 16, 2010 - Upcoming Booster. I got word earlier that Dr. Siwek's office (The Pain Center of Arizona) could get the Ketamine ordered to the apothecary. He will be doing my next set of IV-Ketamine boosters as a trial and if everything goes right, somewhere down the line, he will take other patients needing boosters. I am very excited. Thank you to Dr. Siwek and his staff (especially Michael Hardesty).

I have slowed down a bit on trying new activities. I have to pace myself and do not want to be injured and come out of remission any time soon. How about never? I am getting used to my port, although it does hurt. In addition, the weather changes still really affect me, and it's set to rain two days this coming week. ☹ On February 4, I will be speaking to a fibromyalgia support group on dealing with pain, staying positive, and how to be your best advocate.

February 17, 2010, I get my third set of boosters tomorrow. I am looking forward to it. I have not had the feeling that I "need" to get it, but I am still excited because I want to stay in remission. I am assuming everything will go like the last two times. Dr. Siwek will be performing the infusion here in Peoria,

Arizona. He has a good set-up for his infusion suite. One of the things I must do with the boosters here in Arizona is pick up my own Ketamine. The apothecary shop is holding my case of it and, as I go for an infusion, I pick up the vial for the upcoming booster. I think it is kind of funny, because the pharmacist always asks me if I would like a needle with my Ketamine. I would never try Ketamine at home by myself. I would only do it under supervision. With the side effects of hallucinations and anxiety, without the other medications involved in the process and having lower heart rate during the infusion, I am not comfortable doing it without healthcare professionals present.

The other difference is that Dr. Schwartzman has you take Ativan medication before you arrive. The Versed, Ketamine, anti-nauseous and Clonidine are given to you in your IV bag. With Dr. Siwek, he has me take the Ativan and Clonidine before I arrive. With the drive being over an hour, by the time I get to his office I am out of it and do not really remember or know what is going on, even before we start. Dr. Siwek mixes the Ketamine into the IV solution bag and then puts the Versed and anti-nauseous into a different access point in the

IV line so I get it all at once up front, before the Ketamine starts.

In between the day of boosters, I am out of it. Remember, I am tiny; about 100 lbs. I have other friends who are 200+ lbs. We all get the same dose using Dr. Schwartzman's protocol. Some of them stay awake during the boosters, while I am out of it totally. I do wear a headset with music playing. As they start the Ketamine drip, I always listen to "Bubbly" by Colbie Caillat. It just gives me positive thoughts as I fall asleep. They also told me that during the infusions, if an earpiece falls out, I pout to get the nurses' attention so they can put it back in my ear for me.

My phone is my music player, so I have also texted random strings of letters to my husband and a friend while getting a booster infusion. It is funny because it looks like I am actually making words. I probably have something specific I am saying, but no one would know what I was talking about. After that, I totally get why they do not want you to connect with outside people, especially while in ICU. They say it is because they do not want you to be using your thinking processes. They want the Ketamine to do its job with the least stimuli possible for the best results. I totally understand that and I do see how important it is in the process. However, I am sure it would scare anyone who could not see you and make sure you are okay if they were getting random, non-coherent messages such as this.

March 1, 2010- Third Booster, I got my third set of boosters on February 18th-19th with Dr. Siwek. I got my access line put in on February 17, and the staff at the Scottsdale Healthcare Hospital Infusion Center (Virginia Piper Cancer Center) was very helpful. They remembered me from the access line removal the month before. However, I did not remember a thing from then as I had just finished the infusion with Dr. Siwek. Everything went great with the entire process this time!

The producer from AZTV Ch3 in Phoenix was interviewing Dr. Siwek and me at the start of the first day. The segment should air sometime soon. I am looking forward to seeing it, as I do not remember the taping. Once I find out when the TV interview will air, I will be sure to post it. In addition, I have been asked to do a radio interview this coming Tuesday (March 2) to air on CBS radio called "Sunday Sunrise" with Vicky Carmona. I am excited to be getting so much exposure.

Ken told me I did some funny things. I do not remember any of it, but wanted to share, as the stories are funny to me. First, in the car, on the way home, I was petting a horse. Ken hit a bump in the road and I said he killed the horse. Ken said he was sorry and I said okay and was fine after that, as if nothing had happened. I also asked him if he saw the little people. "Where?" he asked. "Here in the grass," as I was pointing to a "spot of grass" in the car. Then, when we got home, he pulled into the garage. Before he turned off the car, he says, "Okay, are you ready to go home?" I said, "Yes." He turned off the car and said, "We're here." My response: "Boy, was that fast."

The next night after the booster on day two, he took me to a neighbor's house to watch a movie. I slept through the whole thing. However, at one point, the neighbor's dogs started fighting. I sat up and yelled at them to stop, and then fell right back to sleep. Now my neighbors have a funny story about me, too.

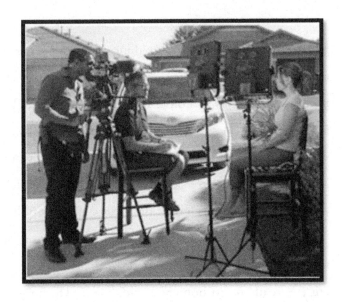

Barby On The Set Of Her Reality Show, Extreme Time Cheaters

IT ALL STARTS AGAIN

Weather changes suck. My pain goes up a couple of days before the storm gets here. The barometric pressure is what is affecting me the most instead of the storms. Either is bad, but before and after is worse than when the storm is directly over me.

April 26, 2010, I am doing a blogtalk.com radio interview with Trudy Thomas from "Living with Hope" tonight. I am really looking forward to being on the air, sharing my knowledge, and advocating for patients. I cannot wait to share my story, tips and tell everyone about my book, *RSD in Me*!

Last week we had a few storms come through here in Arizona. In addition, a little over a week ago, I stepped on a bed rail and it punctured the bottom of my foot. All week I was feeling bad and need to do the IV-Ketamine booster soon. I was also having terrible headaches.

I decided to go to the doctor and get a tetanus shot. The doctor got me in on Saturday morning. I heard that this shot really hurts and was preparing. Well, the nurse used a pediatric needle and it felt smaller than a bug bite. I really did not feel it at all. Then they said that it would hurt worse the next day. So, I prepared for the worst. Well, I think that these people telling me to prepare do not know about pain. Yes, it was achy, but that is it. There was no pain compared to Reflex Sympathetic Dystrophy.

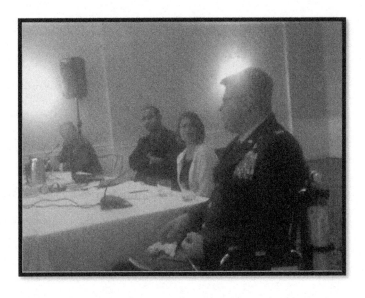

Barby Ingle & Col Douglas Strand, RSD Patients, Testifying at the Department of Defense- Veterans Affairs

Well, I also found out that tetanus has the same neurological symptoms as Reflex Sympathetic Dystrophy; who would have known? It makes me think back and maybe last week I was not doing badly because of the storm, it may have been tetanus. I am feeling like I need to do a Ketamine booster soon; I am going to let my doctor know, so that I can possibly move it up from 20/21 to the 13/14 of May. I hope that will work with Dr. Siwek's schedule.

May 2, 2010, I have decided to get my next booster set early because of the injury when I stepped on a bedrail a few weeks ago. The puncture in the bottom of my foot hurts, as well as burning, swelling, discoloring, etc. It has been bothering me quite a bit. I did end up getting a tetanus shot last weekend and did start to feel better overall after that, but still think it is a good idea to get it early. It will be two weeks early. I will be doing it here in Arizona with Dr. Siwek again. I will get my access line put into my port on Wednesday and then do the IV-Ketamine boosters Thursday and Friday and get the access line taken out Friday afternoon. I am expecting I won't remember anything once again until about Sunday. I am hoping all the pain (yes, I have had a little burning, since hurting my foot), neurological symptoms, and headaches will be gone again.

May 20, 2010, I have come full circle. Just last year I was diagnosed with full body Reflex Sympathetic Dystrophy in Pennsylvania. I was not feeling good at all and the pain was sky high. One year later, I am on the other end of the spectrum.

I am realizing how much I have taken on and it all seems to be coming at me very fast. I am so excited to be doing so well, I want to do everything I can. I just hope my body sticks all the activities out with me. I hope I don't get hurt again. If I do, another IV-Ketamine booster here in Arizona with Dr. Siwek will be in order.

I did not make it to September, let alone a year without incident. It is July and I burnt my hand. I could not get into the doctor right away for an IV-Ketamine booster so I was worried about the booster not being done in time for the procedure to work and would have to start over with the inpatient ICU version. I was trying to do more around the house and I decided to make Ken coffee each morning. I didn't realize that he had already made the coffee and rinsed the pot and put it back on the burner. When I picked up the pot to fill it with water, I saw something on the burner and swiped it. It was an instant burn. The pain had spread up my arm in hours and my body was burning by the next day. I finally got my fifth IV-Ketamine booster (2nd day) July 26/27th and the burning pain went away again. We are still having some storms and monsoons, and there is now just an ache with some electric pains about a level two-three. I am happy to say I am doing well. I know I have to take it easy, not injure myself and keep stress low. I am doing my best.

LIFE DOESN'T GO BACKWARDS

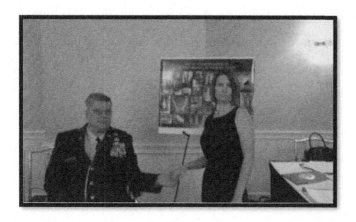

Barby Ingle & Col Douglas Strand, RSD Patients, Testifying at the Department of Defense- Veterans Affairs

As I moved through the last few years, I tried to think about the future and what I wanted to do. It is simple: I want my future to be working, teaching and advocating, so others do not have my past. I am proud of all of my life accomplishments and look forward to this first year to learn my boundaries and set new expectations for the future.

This healthcare system process has taught me that everyone matters. However, the only thing you have control over is how you act and react to challenges. I did not see this before my chronic illness. I mean, I heard it, I said it, but I did not see it, know it or believe it. I am not saying that everyone should get anything they want even if they have not worked hard. In fact, even the most deserving do not always get what they want and some of the least deserving seem to get everything.

Knowing that I am responsible for myself and no matter who I have around to support me or bringing me down, in the end, there is just me. No matter how much you feel entitled to having someone take care of you, because of your illness or whatever other reasons you can think up, it doesn't mean that it is going to happen. For example, just because I am not feeling well I should not be mean or aggressive to someone else. In addition, if I make a choice that affects someone else, they have the right to decide how they deal with it. Just because I want someone to do something doesn't mean they have to or are going to help me. Every action has a reaction. It just may not be what you expect.

As a chronically ill person, I must do what is best for me versus putting guilt on others to do things for me. It is not always the best choice to play the disabled card. At the same time, it is not fair to let yourself sit in pain when you can do something about the situation. Say you are at a dinner party at a family member's house. The host keeps their house cold. That is their right. You can ask them to turn the heat up, but they will not always comply. You have the right to bundle up or leave so that you are doing the best for yourself.

There is more than one side to every story. Just because something appears to be one way does not mean that it is what you perceive. For instance, when you have an invisible illness such as chronic pain, there is something that is wrong, but everything appears to be fine. People do not always know what to say, how to react, or how to help if they were to choose to do something for you. At this point, some patients will choose to say nothing, others will advocate for themselves. It is your choice as to how to react to the challenge. Know that those around you may create assumptions and treat you with behavior that you think is negative. If you just walk away, it may be easier on you now, but in the end, you deal with the stress anyway when resentments build up, patterns form and issues pile on top of issues.

If you have been the type not to "be your own best advocate," it is not too late to start. The good news is that it is not too late. Understand that people who have reacted to you in particular ways may be upset at the moment because change is hard. In the end, you will get better outcomes with the challenge you are overcoming. At the minimum, you will be better off physically and mentally with less negative issues to deal with. What happens when you do not take care of issues? You increase your pain, raise your stress, do not sleep well, and lower your immune system function.

REALISTIC GOALS

My experience has taught me that life goes on. It really does move with or without you. I consciously have chosen to go with what life brings. Some people are stuck in the same mindset they were when the chronic illness happened. For me, that is not the point of living. I am working to have the smartest today so I have the greatest tomorrow. Just because you are dealing with a chronic illness does not take your dignity, respect and living away. It just becomes different. I learned more than ever that I am responsible for myself and that even my husband is not my keeper. Caregivers can only do so much before they need a break, too. You cannot let others fault you, but also be careful not to put guilt on others. Everyone is different and handles the stress of chronic illness differently. Learning this and keeping it in mind has helped me in planning my future.

Looking back, I have been able to complete all of my dreams and life goals set at a young age. I was becoming complacent and not realizing how successful I had become. I was just moving through and looking past the greatness around me. I was not dancing every day, as my dad likes to say. Then I developed Reflex Sympathetic Dystrophy and it was taken away. I realized how much I lost and how far I fell. I went from the top of the world to food stamps and government assistance. It is time I make new dreams, goals, and aspirations. Of course, my body must agree also. I will be working on a new list of life experiences to accomplish.

June 14, 2010, This is just a quick update to let everyone know that things are going well for me. Storms still get me, but I am good. This past Saturday we had a storm and I started to vomit from pain. It was a bad night. The storm left and I am doing better. I found out today that one of my friends is in remission. It is a great day when I get a call that another person is in remission from the burning hell of Reflex Sympathetic Dystrophy. I am glad to be doing well and glad when I hear others are, too. It provides hope to those who are not yet where we are in the healthcare treatment process. I did get my port flushed last week. It was a new nurse, but she did a great job and I did not have any pain from it.

July 15, 2010, we are having many storms roll through the last few days. I am really feeling them and it sucks. I did burn my hand a few weeks ago. Instantly, I had burning in my hand, obviously. Then, it quickly spread to my arm and both legs. I have an IV-Ketamine booster scheduled for July 26th and 27th and, hopefully, it will not be too much time in-between the injury and getting the booster.

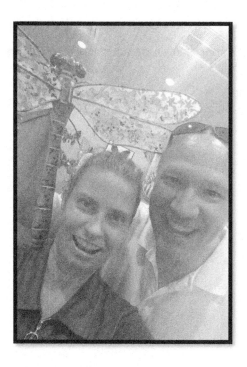

Ken and Barby

Monsoon season is approaching and I am glad to be getting the booster just before. Although, with these storms it feels like it is monsoon season already. This morning I could not get out of bed. Just lying there was painful, too. I was cold, so I wanted to cover up, but then the sheets would hurt so much I tried to stick my legs out. In addition, the part of my back that was very sensitive to touch is back. No giving hugs for a while. I have vomited two times and remain nauseous. My double vision is back, too. It is supposed to be bad weather until Sunday. Yuck! I am looking forward to the upcoming booster.

NO MATTER REMISSION

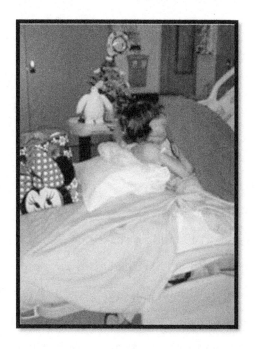

Barby at a Hospital Visit, 2015

With all of the challenges this year, I know that remission does not mean the craziness of Reflex Sympathetic Dystrophy stops. It is okay that I will be dealing with this for life. It is hard. Do not get me wrong. It just is what it is and I have to deal with what I am presented with now. I also have to keep in mind how this moment's decision will influence my future. I have my great days, good days, and poor days. I know that I am not cured by any means. I also know that I am better off than I was a year ago. I am happy to have relief that so many millions of others are still waiting for. Keeping it all in perspective is what I have had to do. I have to look at the milestones from the past year and measure my success from where I was a year before that. I do know that remission is possible; it is just not what I expected.

Now I know the relief of symptoms. Before IV-Ketamine, I would say, "If I could just have one day with no pain it would be a dream." Now I have had many days with no burning pain. I worry about coming out of remission and having to deal with the burning pain everyday non-stop. I worry that the next booster is not going to work. I worry that I am not going to stay trauma-free and my body will revert back permanently. I have to not let it stop me from living. Even before Reflex Sympathetic Dystrophy, I had the attitude of facing my fears and even if I could not conquer it, I could say I did it. Within reason, that is how I am going to live now. I am looking forward and I am going to live to my fullest potential because I do not know when or if it will be here for the rest of my life. I will 'dance' every day.

Now I am out and about town and not taking life for granted as I did before chronic pain. I have been able to go to conferences and doctor appointments without Ken. I have done grocery shopping although manipulating the shopping cart is still difficult and I would not even try it on a bad weather day. When I do get out and do a take on the world activity, by the time I get home, I am tuckered and sometimes have some pains going on. Not normally the burning pain, but more like bone pain, joint pain, sharp pains, and electric pains. My heart races when I go too far or too fast, but I think that has something to do with the port as well as the RSD issue in this case.

I have been able to attend conferences, fly to speak at events around the country and see my family. The freedom is something I missed greatly. I enjoy all of it. I take it easy and keep stress off as much as possible. I travel light, and when alone, have some stranger help me with putting my carry-on bag up and down from the bin on the plane and going through security. They happily do it. I have learned to take breaks more often. Before remission, I was not even able to do activities on a regular basis so these issues were even more challenging.

Now I know that there is a good chance that I will be fine. If I miss a plane because I cannot run to the next gate, it is okay. They put me on the next one. If a bag gets lost or I forget something, it is no big deal. I just let it go; I have to let it go. If I want to do activities that are more regular and last through them this is what I have to do, and so it is. Come what may, I will be okay.

I am hopeful because I have so many friends who are in remission and doing well. I have friends who are on waiting lists and I know they will soon join the the thousands of us who have already benefited from IV-Ketamine infusions. I know that I am helping so many others. This process can be difficult to navigate and there is little instruction on preparing for the treatments and the life of remission. It is not exactly what I expected. I go with the flow and talk to other patients who have done it, and then pass on the knowledge of what happened for them and me to people just starting this process.

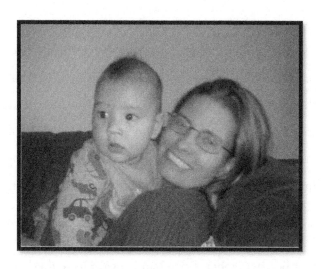

Barby Holding Her Nephew For The First Time

An IV infusion with Ketamine has not worked for all of my friends who have tried it, but it is high percentage in favor of working to some extent and long term. I know people who have done all three levels of the IV-infusions. Some of them have come out of remission, some have been doing well for years and a few it did not help or only helped for a short period. For the ones, it did not help or only helped very short term they had one or both of the following. Either they stayed on their opioids through the process and after, they did not get an initial treatment that was long enough to clear the receptors and have it stick, or both. I also wonder if the ones who do get relief would have better results in a more consistent climate. My friends back East and Midwest have four seasons and barometric pressure rising and falling is a lot more frequent than I have here in Arizona. It would be interesting to see if they come here after a treatment if the relief would be even greater. Can you imagine, all the RSD'ers and people in pain moving to the southwest states for more consistent weather?

For now, I am hopeful that I stay where I am with remission. Get boosters when I need and always have them work. There are no guarantees. Now that I experienced remission, I never want to be put back in the burning hell of full-blown Reflex Sympathetic Dystrophy and all the challenges I went through.

I have been in remission for a year and a few days now. How exciting. I cannot forget that I have relapses. Just the smallest insult to the body can make all the difference in the world. I am so thankful for my doctors, friends, family, Ken and God. Without them, I would not be doing so well.

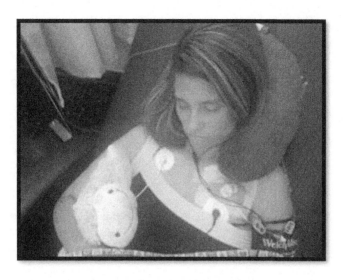

Barby Receiving an Infusion Therapy

Since coming back to Arizona in January 2010, it seems I have taken off with activities. People keep coming to me and asking me to do media projects, speaking engagements and even go back to my cheerleading roots. I am ready to take it all on. I just do not know if my body will always agree. In the first year of remission, I was given opportunities to do so many different events and speaking engagements. I judged a cheerleading competition; testified at the Department of Defense- Veterans Affairs; spoke at Pfizer, Medtronic, American Pain Foundation proceedings and iPain Foundation events around the country. I got to go to American Idol, to Burbank, California for a meeting with show producers, and was able to attend many other organizations events. I testified with my story to get legislation passed for Reflex Sympathetic Dystrophy, step therapy laws, and mandatory pain education classes for healthcare professionals in multiple states. I was in multiple media stories. I loved it all. I do know; however, I took on too much. My body suffered. I must be better at knowing my limits and saying no to all that life has to offer. I am just not ready physically or mentally. Now I know.

KETAMINE INFUSION

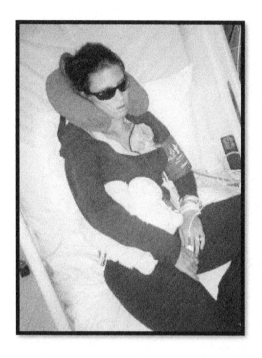

Barby Receiving Infusion Therapy

I get asked this question the most of all of the treatments I have done, so I am going to share. This is information based on my personal treatments as well as many other patient references that I have spoken to over the past 8 years. Keep in mind that every patient is different and your doctor is the one to determine what will work best for you. This is a sample of what works for me and some others.

Pre-K-Infusion

- Testing
- Laboratory
- Cardiac
- Psychological evaluation

Hospital-based infusions

- Five to ten-day in-patient stay
- An intravenous (iv) line is inserted
- Dosing starts at 20mg of Ketamine per hour, which is increased by 5mg increments to a maximum of 40mg per hour
- Clonidine, 0.1 mg (per FDA)
- Lorazepam (Ativan®), 1-to-2 mg, for any dysphoria or hallucinations
- Other medications are utilized to treat such problems as nausea and vomiting, headache etc.

Outpatient protocol

- Initial 10-day outpatient care
- Five days on, 2 off, five days on
- 70mg to 200mg of Ketamine per day in titrating doses over the 10 days and then start the outpatient booster program
- Most patients are given 2 mg of Midazolam and sleep through the procedure
- Other medications are given as needed for side effects such as nausea and headache

Booster Protocol

- Following discharge from the hospital or 10-day outpatient care, patients enroll in an outpatient infusion booster program
- The booster program consists of two consecutive outpatient treatments a week every other week for one month, then two consecutive treatments one month later, then two consecutive treatments at three months.
- Outpatient visits are then monthly, or at 3-month intervals. This is done in two or more consecutive days. Exact protocol depends on the patient and varies at

times.

- Barby's outpatient dose of Ketamine is 200mg each day.

ORAL ORTHOTIC

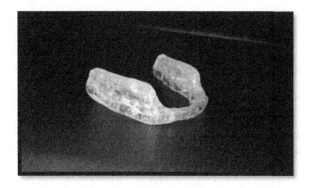

Barby's Oral Orthotic

Over the years, I have participated in many research studies and up-and-coming potential treatment options. One of the studies was published in 2016 in the Journal of Translational Medicine by doctors Garabed G. Demerjian, Andre Barkhordarian and Francesco Chiappelli.

So many people over the years meet me and soon realize that I have a device called an oral orthotic in my mouth. This OO as I lovingly call it has given me so much on a practical daily level. Now there is published science behind what it is doing for me. I know what it does and how much better my life has become but to be able to be a part of studies that have helped change my life for the better is amazing. To know that this work will help so many more patients long after me is even more exciting. The traditional research in the health sciences has involved control and experimental groups of patients, and descriptive and inferential statistical analyses performed on the measurements obtained from the samples in each group. This research I was part of was a novel model of translation healthcare. The novel model of translational healthcare integrates translational research and translational effectiveness. This type of research is increasingly becoming more established in modern contemporary medicine.

I often say that each patient is different. Our biological makeup and life experiences makes the same disease affect us in a variety of ways that makes one size medicine approach impractical. Science is seeing this too. The research that the doctors above and others like them are doing focus broadly on translational research for the ultimate benefit of each individual patient. This is what we need.

What the research was like from the patient perspective. These research doctors and my treating doctor, Dr. G Demerjian approached this with an individualized approach that they made measurable for each of us in the study. I underwent multiple fMRI, cat-scans, X-rays, synovial fluid testing, psychological testing, and saliva testing. These tests were done to quantify the outcome and show the effectiveness of the oral orthotic use. I underwent this study in 2015 but first received my OO in 2012. I knew from what it had done for me that the tests were going to show amazing results. That is great for the scientific community and advancing a new treatment options for others. For me, the proof came when I was fitted for my first OO December 2012.

Now for what the Oral Orthotic has done for me on a practical level. The first thing I notice was my vision. Back in 2002 when I developed reflex sympathetic dystrophy I lost partial vision in my right eye. I saw many eye doctors and ENT doctors who were unable to pinpoint where the breakdown in the nerves were. They hypothesized that it was due to inflammation from the RSD cutting off a pathway. Within 30 seconds of putting in the OO I had my vision back after 10 years of being told that I would never have it back. My world is now brighter with the OO, literally.

I also have had improvement in my pain levels affecting my entire body. You could never imagine that the pain in your foot could be caused by neuroinflammation. This showed me exactly how it is all connected. I have been able to get my infusion therapy minimized to only 1-2 boosters a year and get off all daily pain medication. I also have had improvement in my balance, coordination, dystonia, memory and mood. My migraines and headaches are less often and although weather and pressure changes still affect me, it is not to the extent it was prior to my Oral Orthotic use.

I know and understand that being part of a research study is not for everyone and doesn't always go as great as it has for me. Seeing how stepping up and trying something that not many others are doing has helped not only my life but many others to come is so rewarding. The process is not always seen from the patient perspective, but working with the providers with the approach that they took to create and develop a way to measure scientifically the benefits that those of us as patients can experience first-hand has been an amazing process. I thank all the research doctors and scientists who are out there making a difference in our lives. I know it can take years to see what you are working on come to market. When it comes time to share with the world the difference you are making in our lives I find it hard to express the gratitude to the magnitude that you have given back to millions. Thank you to our researchers in the chronic pain community.

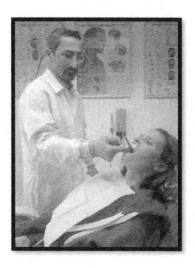

Barby Being Fitted for an Oral Orthotic By Dr. Demerjian

FEELINGS

Mental health can be disrupted when living with a chronic pain disease. Anxiety, depression, feeling of hopelessness, isolation and helplessness can increase to dangerous levels. Particularly for people who have been suffering with chronic pain for a long period, life can become overwhelming. When I finally realized that RSD had no cure and that my future would include pain daily, I began to have dark thoughts. I do not want to end up at the risk of suicide. There are going to be good and bad days, and if this is a bad day for you, remember to focus on the good days, good feelings and positive past and future experiences. It is very important for you and your family to recognize the symptoms of diminished emotional well-being and act.

Understand that these feelings and thoughts are common among chronic pain'ers. It is helpful to create an overall strategy to get through the rough times. Chronic pain patients learn over time that they can better cope and adjust to both the physical and psychological consequences of the disorder with the help and support of spiritual guidance, family and therapists. Creating an arsenal of tools, such as spirituality, physical modalities and meditation, are all ways to better your situation. Turning to God has especially helped me with anxiety, depression and other psychological / physical challenges, and it offers a great way to cope with and put situations into proper perspective so we can learn to live with it.

Chronic pain is not understood very well, and there are physicians and psychiatrists who believe that it is all in our heads or that people just complain for the sake of workmen's compensation issues. If we are malingering patients who just won't go away, doctors who don't understand chronic pain may find it difficult to look for any other diagnosis other than psychological. A lot of my stress could have been avoided if doctors had really listened to me from the start instead of looking at my marriage troubles as an excuse to "be ill for attention."

With the loss of independence and function, it is hard for many patients to accept their changing life. Be sure to surround yourself with a team who is on your side, or you will be in a fight in which you will have trouble winning. I went through a grieving process during coming to grips with my new reality. This is not uncommon for chronic pain patients.

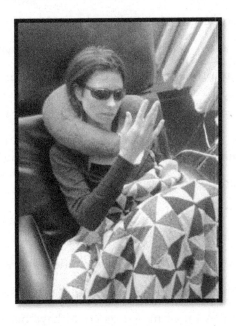

Barby During Infusion Therapy, Discovering a Pain Free Hand

There were stages to my grieving. First was hope. I hoped that there was some cure to make the pain go away. Second, wondering if the treatment I was receiving was appropriate, I got angry. The feeling of resentment and depression from when I realized that this is not temporary is sometimes overwhelming. When this happens, I try to rationalize and evaluate the changes in my life and how I live it. In doing this I come to an understanding and acceptance of what my place is with the permanent pain.

It is important that patients with chronic pain and other chronic pain conditions maintain a healthy lifestyle, including getting enough sleep, exercising, and eating healthy foods, despite the difficulties we experience. There are long-term health consequences created by our changing lifestyle because of chronic pain. As patients with chronic pain, we typically lead a more sedentary lifestyle due to our pain. Because we are less active, we are at greater risk for developing other medical problems. I myself have been dealing with poor posture and sudden weight gain and loss. I fall easily and have trouble gripping and holding onto things. In the long-term, we need to watch out for cardiovascular disease, diabetes and osteoporosis as the risk for these conditions is heightened with inactivity.

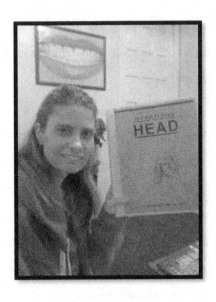

Barby at a Doctor's Office Waiting to Be Seen

Weight control is my biggest issue. As a former athlete, I know it is crucial for good health. Nutrition also plays a role in chronic pain and how we prepare our bodies to cope with the stress on us every day. Make sure that your doctor is doing frequent blood testing to check for any deficiencies you may develop. Medications can also affect your liver, kidneys and digestive system. Blood testing can help prevent this from getting out of control as well as let you know if there are any vitamin supplements you may need to take to counter poor absorption. Try finding clubs and workout facilities that offer programs for physically handicapped individuals, or use things around your house if you do not get out often, as is the case for me.

I try to use my affected arm as much as possible. I tend to shield my arm from any stimulation and from being touched or manipulated due to the increase in pain levels, even from the smallest of stimuli. This is something to overcome and find solutions around. For instance, my caretakers assist me in bathing and other activities that are painfully overwhelming for me. Maintaining good hygiene may be painful but is very important. My new reality is that I am disabled and do need to ask for help. This is also part of a cycle. Every new doctor, therapist and even talk of a new treatment from other patients gives me that hope once again. I now understand that healing is a process, and I have control with how I look at life my life. The cycle of grief is shown through anger, resentment, depression, understanding, hope and then acceptance.

I have found that patients with chronic pain, including myself, experience depression, fear, anxiety and anger. The idea of living with this horrible syndrome with no cure is astounding. A study by the International Association for the Study of Pain recommends that psychological intervention be initiated for patients experiencing pain for more than two months.[7] When my experience with chronic pain started, I was already in therapy for personal reasons, but it soon became apparent that my nameless symptoms were taking over my life, and I was unable to focus on anything but coping with "the new me." When doctors told me, "Just do this and you will be okay," I would build up my hope and follow their directions. When I did not get better, I came crashing down, and so did life around me. I have since gone to therapy on and off throughout my process of learning to live with chronic pain. I tried group therapy and found it to be better than one-on-one counseling for me. Hearing that I was not the only one out there in this large world gave me a peace.

Relaxation and meditation techniques, I had learned in my sessions help me reduce muscle spasms, pain, and improve my dysfunctional sleeping patterns. Learning to LIVE with pain and still accomplish life goals is an important part of treatment. Counseling helps me cope, raises my self-esteem and prepares

---

[7] Physical Medicine and Rehabilitation Review, Pg 179, International Association for the Study of Pain, Contributor Robert J. Kaplan, Published by McGraw-Hill, 2005

me mentally to take on chronic pain instead of allowing chronic pain to take me. Having positive thoughts, even self-given, helps me remain positive and change my behavior and emotional state.

This biofeedback is a way to train our bodies to improve our health. We can use signals both visually and auditory from our own bodies to improve our condition. This is a powerful tool that gives us some choice in our reaction to our pain. Biofeedback can also help with blood pressure, heart rate, muscle tension and body temperature, which all contribute to our chronic pain. Many doctors report better outcomes with patients who use this biofeedback technique. Lowering anxiety and fear and the ability to relax through the tough times help us cope better with the chronic pain. Practicing coping techniques like meditation, deep breathing, visual imaging, yoga and other such relaxing activities daily will help us improve our pain control. This improvement will allow us to be in command of our own life as well as reduce our pain levels.

Calming the mind and body through mental relaxation will improve our function; we just should do it consistently and effectively. I have found that keeping a positive attitude helps me cope with the pain as well as the daily stresses in life. Adopting positive thinking as a way of life can help lower the pain levels as well as help you with stress and anxiety-filled situations. When I am in a stressful situation or face a life challenge, I find it brings constructive changes if I look at the situation in an optimistic light. Optimism is confidence, hopefulness and a cheerful way of coping with a challenge that is seemingly daunting. To me, optimism is believing that things are continually getting better and that good will ultimately prevail over evil.

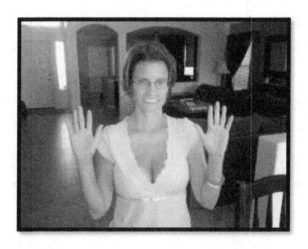

Barby Showing Her Finger Can Straighten After Infusion Therapy

Creating a positive attitude starts with being inspired. Begin by finding an interest or hobby you can become involved with and will enjoy. A few suggestions are joining a non-profit cause, solving puzzles, writing a journal, joining or starting a support group, or even starting a blog. Creating a purpose can assist with your self-esteem and confidence. Just because you are disabled does not mean you are not worth anything. I have learned that every person has a value no matter how big or small. Believing in yourself and in your abilities, choosing happiness and thinking creatively is good motivation when it comes to accomplishing your goals. Expect success when you are going through your daily activities. It might take you longer or you may need to use more constructive thinking to achieve success, but it is possible.

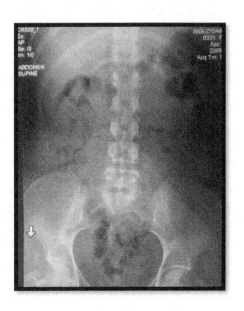

X-ray of Barby with Ischemia and Severe OIC

Negative situations are bound to appear, but when you are looking for solutions and displaying self-esteem and confidence, you will also attract other people to participate in helping you accomplish your needs and goals. Try looking at failure and problems as blessings in disguise. Doing so will help solutions find you. Seize the opportunities in everyday life. Using your outings to inform others of your condition, finding pleasure in your minor accomplishments, and not giving up are just a few ways to increase your power of positive thinking.

There are great benefits to having a positive attitude. Especially when things are not going your way, staying optimistic will allow you more energy, happiness and lower pain levels. Achieving goals is a great motivator for positive thinking. Success is achieved faster and more easily through positive thinking, and it will inspire and motivate you and others. I have found that when I am letting the pain get the better of me, it comes across to others as disrespect and brings those around me down.

Staying calm and positive creates an atmosphere for greater inner strength and power. You can also create better communication with a calm positive attitude, which will assist you in working with your doctors and caretakers. When you take life one task at a time and approach each challenge with optimism, it leads to fewer difficulties encountered along the way and increases the ability to overcome any difficulty. As my father always says when I am having a bad day, "Tomorrow will be a better day."

No matter the challenges of today, they will pass, and in retrospect, they will not seem as bad as time moves on. The challenges may just turn out to be a bump that looked like a mountain at the time. Remez Sasson says, "Positive attitude helps us to cope more easily with the daily affairs of life. It brings optimism into your life, and makes it easier to avoid worry and negative thinking.

If you adopt it as a way of life, it will bring constructive changes into your life, and makes them happier, brighter and more successful."[8] I have found that when I live life with a negative attitude I am saying that I do not respect myself and do not believe success is possible. Try working on displaying a positive attitude and the moods of others and the challenges of life will become easier to deal with. Choosing to be happy starts with you. No person or thing can make you happy and positive. It is a skill you must practice and develop when living with chronic pain. When you can live in a happy, positive and optimistic light, your life will become a life worth the ups and downs that come with it.

---

[8] The Power of Positive Attitude, Remez Sasson, successconsciousness.com

WHAT DO YOU SAY

You can never take back information once it is shared but you can always wait to let people know later. If you choose to disclose that you have chronic pain, decide when and how to do so. If there is time to prepare ahead of time, it is a good idea. Take time to think about different situations and how you wish to handle them.

Many people feel it is not their place to ask about your physical conditions, but knowing about chronic pain and chronic pain would help them understand where you are coming from with your thoughts and actions. When you are deciding to disclose your chronic pain and limitations, make the decision whether to let others know about your invisible disability.

I know a chronic pain patient who liked a neighbor and was interested in dating him. He often helped around her house with handyman projects, and she would see him out on his porch and go out and talk to him. Eventually, he asked her out, and they had a great time. Over the next few months they had dates scheduled but she ended up canceling a lot of them.

She was just in too much pain. He began to think she was not interested in him and started to pull away. Friends encouraged her to tell him about RSD and what she is going through. She did, and he stuck around for a while. In the end, it did not work out. They remained friends and it helped her see that you can still have a social life despite the chronic pain.

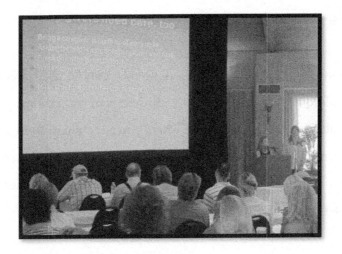

Barby Doing A Presentation To Other Pain Patients

If you're in this or another social situation you should think about the following when deciding to disclose your chronic pain and how it affects your everyday life. Are you able to participate in the activities at hand using your coping skills and tools? Do you need accommodations? Are you able to perform the activity safely if you choose not to disclose?

Secondly, do you think they will react in a way appropriate for the environment you are in? If you are not sure, you may want to wait until you are in a private setting. If the situation becomes an intimate relationship, it is important to share even if it means losing the person. It is not fair to them or yourself to keep information back. If your disability is in remission or typically under control, is there a reason to disclose? Possibly the education you give them may help someone else they meet along the way. It is possible that flare-ups on your part may keep you from future activities.

Finally, how will you address misconceptions about your disability when you disclose? Some people do not believe in treating pain with narcotic medications or have a bad experience with someone else in their life with chronic pain. Having them not understanding can lead to a divide. Also, not telling others is not an option if you are in a situation that can cause others harm. For instance, when getting on a plane, you cannot have the exit row. If assigned by mistake, notify the flight crew.

When choosing situations and activities where you do not want to disclose your disability, take time to carefully analyze the kind activities you can do and plan accordingly. Remember, you can always reveal more information later as needed.

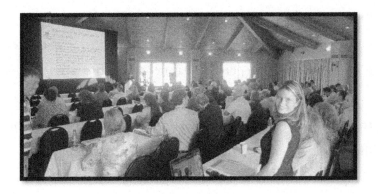

Barby About to do Her Presentation for a Group of Pain Patients

Too many people misinterpret chronic pain. There are many physicians who are not familiar with the condition and its symptoms, and many who perceive their patients' complaints to be psychiatric in nature ("it's all in your head"). In addition, since chronic pain is related to many cases of workmen's compensation for injury occurring on the job or personal injury cases, there may be a tendency for some health care providers to view the patient's complaints as malingering. This is a significant source of stress for many patients, including myself, and may lead to significant delays in diagnosis and treatment. This situation adds to the psychosocial issues that we as patients already deal with due to chronic pain. It can disrupt quality of life and treatments.

As a patient, you may have to deal with a loss of independence as your level of functioning may be significantly compromised. It is hard for many patients to accept their changing condition. Many go through a grieving process during coming to grips with their new reality.

Some medical literature describes seven stages through which people move in relating to chronic pain including:[9]

- Acceptance & hope
- Anger & bargaining
- Depression, reflection, loneliness
- Pain & guilt
- Reconstruction & working through
- Shock & denial

_____

[9] 7 Stages of Greif, Through the Process and Back to Life, recover-from-grief.com

- The upward turn

As a pain patient, I have gone through the stages of grief with a slightly different perspective. I wondered if the treatment I was receiving was appropriate. I had, and still have, hope that there will someday be a cure. I did have feelings of anger, resentment and was depressed when I realized that the pain was not temporary. I finally coped by evaluating the changes in my lifestyle as I learned to accept that permanent pain and varying levels of disability were part of my new reality.

Family and friends who form the support group around the patient must be educated and aware of the fluid nature of chronic pain. Fluid meaning that symptoms come and go, the patient might be up one minute and down the next, have a fever, sweating, swelling, discoloration and the like and then it settles down until the next flare-up. If the caretakers learn the possible treatment and rehabilitation options, patient's behaviors that should be encouraged or discouraged, and take the supporting role, the family and patient will better communicate with each other. It is very important for friends and family to try to understand what the patient is going through and allow the patient the opportunity to express his or her emotions. Patients need to feel that they can show their grief and frustration without being judged by their supporters. I am lucky to have family and friends who are supportive and encourage me to keep my spirits up and to continue functioning to the best of my ability.

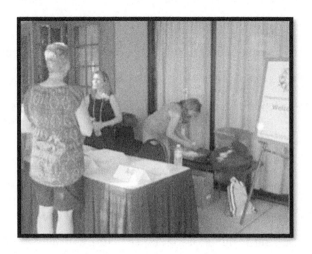

Barby Helping with Registration at a Pain Conference

Not all treatments work for all chronic pain patients. Pushing different treatment modalities is harmful to the communication process. Like me, patients get tired of being "lab rats." Although making suggestions is a positive behavior for a family member or friend, do not get discouraged as a supporter if the patient chooses something else or had tried what you suggested and it did not work for them.

Some patients become depressed if their condition prevents them from doing things that are important to their independence and well-being. I was an independent person who had to learn how to rely on others for daily tasks (e.g., dressing, cooking, and errands). This is not only inconvenient, but can lead to feeling worthless and can be demeaning. Having independence taken away tends to rob patients of their self-respect. It is important to address these feelings and to respond appropriately as a supporter. Attitude and self-perception are crucial factors for continuing to maintain a good quality of life. As patients struggle with their situation, they may be having feelings of inadequacy and worthlessness. You can encourage them to be social and participate in life activities through positive communication.

From my experiences, I would suggest that a patient be encouraged to join a support group or to seek psychological counseling, if appropriate. Be sure to find a support group that focuses on a positive patient life and social skills. Patients may even reach the point of mentoring and counseling others with chronic pain. Some patients find benefit in getting involved in volunteer work. Volunteering allows them to set their own hours and to feel that they can still contribute to others instead of just focusing on their own condition.

Despite a wide range of treatment options available to patients with chronic pain, some patients do not seek help. Patients may be discouraged from reaching out by constant pain. They are worn down both physically and emotionally. This may result in dismissing support and effort from others to help them. Some patients are concerned with fears. Fear that nothing can help them or that the side effects from treatments will be too much to handle. They fear that they will become addicted to the medications or they will develop a tolerance to medications and the recurring pain will be even worse. Patients often hear that they are "complainers" if they talk about their pain, so a fear of communication can develop.

It is important for the patient to discuss these concerns with family members, friends, physicians, and support service professionals (e.g., psychologist, social worker) to take advantage of options that are available. These options may lead to pain relief and improvement in the overall quality of their life. Helping them through the fear makes the whole process easier on them.

LOSING TO MANY FRIENDS

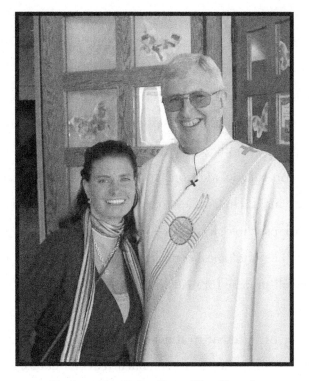

Barby with a Priest From Her Church

I wanted to touch on this subject because I have lost many friends over the years as their pain was not properly treated in a timely manner. Many others I have met have contemplated suicide or attempted it without success. Because currently there is no cure for most chronic pain diseases, the disorder may persist for a prolonged period and can have a significant psychosocial impact on patients. The chronic, severe nature of pain experienced by many chronic pain patients, particularly those with established and long-standing chronic pain, may lead to psychological co-morbidity, including anxiety, feelings of isolation, depression, and a sense of hopelessness and helplessness. In some cases, the adverse psychological consequences of the chronic pain may increase the risk of suicide or suicide ideation. It is, therefore, important for patients and their families to recognize and understand the potential psychological effects of chronic pain and seek a thorough psychological consultation and evaluation as part of the overall strategy for managing chronic pain.

A variety of different treatment options are available to help chronic pain patients with concurrent psychological co-morbidity, including drug therapy and cognitive behavior therapy. A multidisciplinary approach to treatment involving a pain management specialist, neurologist, physiatrist (specialist in physical medicine and rehabilitation), and a psychologist or psychiatrist may be necessary to help chronic pain patients learn to better cope and adjust to both the physical and psychological consequences of the disorder.

Your attitude and self-perception are crucial factors for continuing to maintain a good life. As I struggle with my situation with sometimes, feelings of inadequacy and worthlessness, I find it beneficial to keep a journal, set realistic goals, attend church, learn and read. I use these tools to increase my knowledge of myself as well as gain useful knowledge about the chronic pain in me and to grow stronger spiritually.

All humans experience pain. Like me, many people spend time trying to find something in our spirituality that offers an escape from our pain. Pain is part of our reality, humanity and responsibility. Understanding that not all pain is bad is important in this process. As humans, we need pain to keep us from danger and lead us to responsible activities that prolong our race and ourselves.

Chronic pain is bad pain. Pain becomes bad when it outstays its usefulness. When you have bad pain, it is just that: bad pain. Trying to ignore it is harmful to us and to society. Bad pain must be dealt with as it affects our spirituality and our willingness to carry on humanity and our responsibility to God.

Often, we ask ourselves, "Is somehow having chronic pain a way for God to test my strength?"

Pain is often associated with suffering. Does our suffering improve our ability to help humanity? At one point or another, my pain has affected my creativity and has caused chaos when not put into perspective. Many people make a choice to move closer to God or close Him out when a chronic condition affects them directly. For me, I have found a deeper awareness of God's presence in my life and in those around me. I choose to look at the world through positivism and miracles. There are dark times in most chronic pain sufferers' paths where we contemplate what we are here for. Finding a goal and the path to follow is important to keeping up our spirits. Without goals and direction, we tend to create disharmony and chaos. If we are not aware of God in our life, our pain loses its humanity. To stop LIVING would be the worst thing we could do to get through the pain. Turning to our higher power and using our worldly tools will help us achieve for the greater good of everyone.

Through physical activity, we LIVE and pick up our spirits. Remembering to keep within my appropriate level of exercising or physical movement, every now and then, I push myself a little beyond to see if I have made any gains. I usually end up paying for it the next few days, but I am glad to have made it through the test and know where my new boundaries lie.

My spirituality has really come into play with my physical abilities as well. Many days and nights, I pray that I will make it through another successful activity. I believe the saying, "God only gives you what you can handle." However, I also wish He did not think I could handle so much. The fact that I am LIVING and handling the pain is a testament to my faith and my abilities I did not know I had.

Pain is ultimately a mystery to us all. Sometimes nothing can be done about the causes of chronic pain in our life. When I have no choices, and am only pain-filled, believing that we are the body of Christ and the final glory will be in all, the pain becomes more bearable for me. My suffering leads to the suffering of all involved in my life. It takes a toll on all of us because of our inability to know what to do.

When I am in severe pain, I try to share the pain experience with others, not to complain, but to find understanding, despite knowing deep down that we can never feel what someone else's pain is like.

As we encounter pain, we become stronger in faith or weaker in faith. Pain can destroy a person and those around him. If you allow it, pain will destroy everything good in your life. Those of us who live a life of unsought pain represent the mystery of life and our deep need for survival as a race.

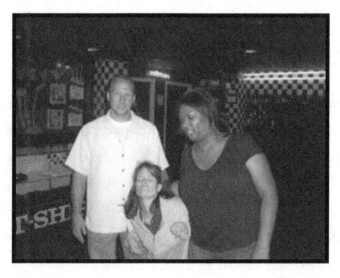

After Being Touch Unexpectedly, I React Instinctively To The Pain

My spirituality has grown from my need for survival. My daily prayer and hope is to lessen the pain. As the pain transforms me, my instinct for survival, which is a deep instinct for us all, strengthens me and helps me stay in the light of God's grace.

OPPORTUNITIES

There is no cure for most chronic pain disease, but progress is being made to find the underlying process of developing chronic pain in many of the diseases that have been identified to date. If we can understand this process, then options to cure diseases involving chronic pain may come about more rapidly. The earlier we catch and properly treat what is causing the chronic pain, the better the chances for that patient to have a good outlook in controlling the chronic pain or putting it into remission. If the symptoms and pain progresses and is not addressed or is incorrectly treated, the issues become more complex and invasive.

It is important to learn about the types of treatments available to you either through insurance coverage or cash pay. Treatment options include physical therapy, medication, orthopedic surgery, invasive surgery, non-invasive procedures, naprapathy, stem cell therapy, infusion therapy, and literally hundreds of other options. Patients should look for ways to control and minimize pain and discomfort to the greatest extent possible. Coping skills will develop out of necessity with chronic pain patients. However, we sometimes need to speak to someone on the outside of our circle for a different view. Psychological counseling may become necessary. It is okay to ask for help when needed.

Goal creation and treatment plans should also include: drug management, family/social adjustment, improvement of the patient's quality of life and psychosocial functioning, and increasing mobilization or range of motion through physical therapy to help prevent progression and aggravation of symptoms. It is important to treat the underlying symptoms even if it means turning to surgical intervention in some cases. Depending on how well you respond to the various options, a progression of treatments will be determined by your team of providers and yourself as an engaged and empowered patient. Remember you as the patient needs to play an important and vocal role in creating the plan.

Accomplishing the goals of treating your chronic pain begins with patient awareness. Setting goals and a timetable that is reasonable can be done with your providers. On my good days I try a few new activities and increase the amount of physical activity as able. By doing this I have seen an increase in my body functioning, range of motion, muscle strength, improve balance and posture.

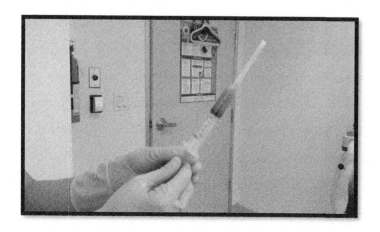

Barby's Stem Cells About to Be Put into Her IV Bag

For me, as the pain increases, I find myself slouching more. Becoming aware of yourself and your environment greatly increases your chances of successful treatment of chronic pain and a better quality of life. Get involved in movement training. This can include walking for two minutes at a time or, if you're ambitious, a mile. Do what you can do at your level. It will be different for all of us. Moving will increase your health and the function of your body, and it also helps with constipation and gastrointestinal issues caused by the chronic pain and medications. Movement increases your blood circulation, which helps with atrophy and can decrease hypersensitivity.

Using a combined therapy approach can give you faster relief. When most people think of physical therapy they think of machines and weights. However, I learned that there are many types of therapy that fall under the same realm of "physical". These therapies are more in line with what we can handle. The other physical therapy methods include biofeedback, hot compresses, elevation, massage, range of motion exercises, and hydrotherapies. There is some thought that physical therapy is painful and does not help. Patients can combine counseling, physical therapy and a drug regimen for better relief. Doing this can help us stay on track with our treatment plan and increase the benefits of physical therapy. Again, it comes back to surrounding yourself with a team of doctors, caretakers, and family supporters that have the education on chronic pain to support you.

The good news is that no matter how long you have had chronic pain you can be helped in some way, if you are willing to stay active, can avoid unnecessary surgical procedures, can change medication usage when appropriate and will improve nutrition and posture habits. Unfortunately, chronic pain affects many systems of the body over time, the autonomic and central nervous system, immune system, limbic, gastrointestinal and more.

The treatments that helped me the most were iv infusion therapy with Ketamine, my own personal stem cells, Alignmed Posture apparel, Oral Orthotic, and aqua therapy.

Some of the other treatments I have done over the years are:

- Acupressure
- Aromatherapy
- Art Therapy
- Calmare
- Chiropractic
- Creative visualization
- Energy medicine
- Holistic living
- Home remedies
- Hydrotherapy
- Journaling
- Ketamine Infusions
- Laser light therapy
- Medication: Opioids
- Medication: NSAIDS
- Medication: (other)
- Massage therapy
- Meditation
- Mindfulness
-

- Music therapy
- Naturopathic medicine
- Nerve block
- Nutritional diet
- Oral Orthotics
- Physical Therapy
- Pilates
- Posture Apparel
- Prayer
- Radio frequency ablation
- Reflexology
- Spinal Epidural Blocks
- Stem Cell Infusions
- Supplements
- Support groups
- Therapeutic touch
- Trigger point injections
- Vitamin therapy
- Yoga

Some of the procedures I have had include:

- 1998- Laparoscopy, Endometriosis
- 1999 - Hysterectomy, Endometriosis, (Also Left Ovary & Appendix at the Same Time)
- 2001 - Right Knee Surgery, Torn Meniscus and MCL
- 2003 - Right Shoulder Surgery
- 2003 - Right Rib Resection, Thoracic Outlet Syndrome
- 2003 - Right Lung Tube Insertion, Due to TOS Surgery Complication
- 2004 - Right Rib Resection, Thoracic Outlet Syndrome
- 2004 - Oral Surgery
- 2005 - Stint Put in For Removal Of Kidney Stone
- 2005 - 2008 - Radiofrequency Procedure Every 5-7 Weeks, Reflex Sympathetic Dystrophy Treatment
- 2007 - Gastrectomy Upper/Lower- Bleeding Ulcers
- 2009 - IV Ketamine Infusion, Inpatient
- 2010 - IV Ketamine Infusion Boosters (Approx. Every 3 Months)
- 2011 – Upper/Lower GI, For Bleed, Kidney Stones, IV Ketamine Infusion
- 2012 – Kidney Stones, IV Ketamine Infusion, Dec – got Oral Orthotic

- 2013 – Kidney Stones, Gall Bladder Removal, Upper/Lower GI, For Bleed, IV Ketamine Infusion
- 2014 - Upper/Lower GI, For Bleed ischemia, IV Ketamine Infusion
- 2015 - Upper/Lower GI, For Bleed ischemia, Kidney Stones, Heart Ischemia & Backflow, Stem Cell Infusion, IV Ketamine Infusion
- 2016 –Broken Foot, Stem Cell Infusion with ketamine, Hospitalization: Lactic buildup

And finally, some of the diagnoses in my medical history:

- Anemia
- Arthritis
- Asymmetry of the Hypothalamus
- Blood Chemistry Abnormalities
- Chronic Ischemia (intestines and heart)
- Colitis
- Colon Polyps
- Depression, Situational, Recurrent
- Dystonia
- Endometriosis
- Finger Fracture
- Foot Fracture
- Gallstones
- Horner's Syndrome
- Hypothyroidism
- IBS
- Kidney Stones
- Medial Meniscus Tear
- Oral Tumors
- Reactive Airway Disease
- Reflex Sympathetic Dystrophy/Central Pain Syndrome
- Seizure Disorder
- TMJ Disease
- Toe Fracture
- Traumatic Ecchymosis
- Tricuspid Insufficiency
- Vertigo

BUT YOU LOOK SO GOOD

At this point, there is no cure, only remission. Very few chronic pain patients ever go into remission, but it is possible. In the meantime, you can do some things to make life more enjoyable and bearable. Start by finding the right doctor, test out the pain medicines and procedures that you are comfortable with, and communicate with your doctors, caretakers and family to create a treatment plan that works for you.

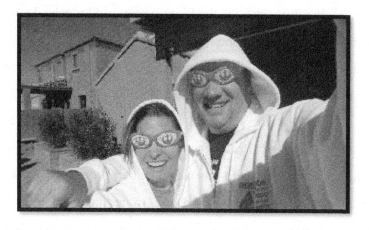

Ken and Barby Dressing Up for NERVEmber

I found that the people who were your friends before chronic pain tend to not handle the thought of you never getting better very well. Lose the people in your life who are not supporting you, whether that person is a doctor or a friend since first grade; you do not need their stress. Your emotional well-being is just as important as finding relief from the pain. I keep track, in a journal, of when pain is stronger, of when symptoms flare, and of general life experiences. I find this helpful in making sure that I am getting the right treatment and that I am not making myself worse.

Remember, for some, the medications you need to take do not have to be of a strong dosage; take what you need for maximum relief and life function. I am using the method of taking the minimum so that I do not build up a tolerance too quickly. Since there is no cure for chronic pain yet, I want to stretch out what I do have available for relief. After working and communicating with other chronic pain patients who have had chronic pain for at least ten years more than me, I see that it can get worse; it can spread, and it can be more pain than you have today, if you can imagine that. Getting the word out, educating people and lobbying for additional research and awareness is our best hope of ending the pain.

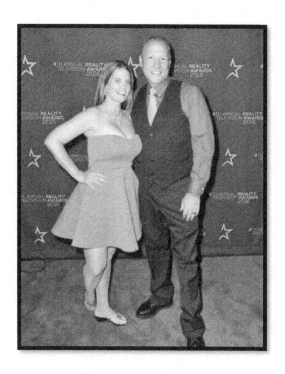

Ken and Barby at the Reality TV Awards

When looking for the right doctor to work with you, one who is willing to work with you to treat the chronic pain in you, ask the important questions. Are there any doctors in my area who specialize in managing chronic pain patients? You can check with local chronic pain support groups and ask the doctors if they have a chronic pain patient that they are currently treating or have treated in the past so you can speak with them. There are activities you can be doing on your own. You can improve your condition or at least prevent it from getting worse. Keep in mind that with chronic pain, pain equals no gain. You should not take an athletic mentality or approach to dealing with your chronic pain. Ask your current/potential doctor, how much experience they have had treating patients with chronic pain. Does that doctor feel there is one treatment that is better than others or that they are more comfortable performing?

In choosing treatments, I have run into situations with insurance companies where they do not cover the treatment I wish to have. My husband's company seems to change insurers each year, and every insurer has covered different things or needed the treatments coded in a specific way so that they will cover it. It is a good idea to find out what your health insurance policy will cover before treatment is administered.

Every patient is different and responds differently with treatments. Find out what the doctor thinks your short term and long-term prognosis looks like. Create a team of health care professionals. Find out what types of healthcare professionals your doctor thinks should be involved in your treatment. When a treatment is suggested, find out why. What are the pros and cons to the recommendation?

Remember, be the Chief of Staff of your medical team. You oversee you, and it is your responsibility to investigate from multiple sources before making a treatment decision that may affect your future. Just because something takes the pain away today does not make it the best option for your future. Ask if the side effects can be reversed and if there are chances of any lasting negative complications prior to any invasive procedure.

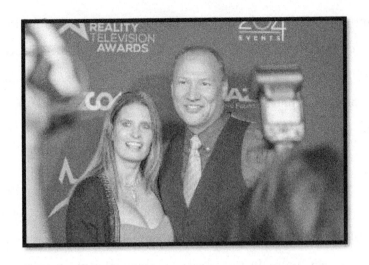

Ken and Barby at the Reality TV Awards Red Carpet

One of the hardest things of this chronic illness for me has been the inability to work a sustainable job. Until it was gone from my life, I did not realize how important work was. Work provides a financial stability but also helps our sense of purpose. Having a purpose, or a sense of being needed, gave me a self-esteem boost and a better quality of life. One of the biggest things that helped me emotionally after chronic pain was finding things that I could do to help others. Although I received my degree in social psychology, my life was focused and prepared around cheerleading, dance and gymnastics. I did not train for anything else; I had no fall back plan. It was hard for me to go from working nonstop to being inactive. That is what chronic pain can do to you. I lost a lot of friends, and my social life became nonexistent. One therapy to think about when you are in this situation is occupational therapy. This is an important step in gaining back and seeing new ways to be an active and productive member of society. With chronic pain, you must become creative in your everyday life situations. If you need someone to cut your food so it is easier to eat, you could return the favor by first thanking them and then offering to do something that you can do, like tutor their child in math or read them a book.

FINAL THOUGHTS

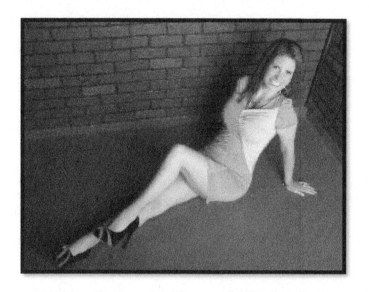

Barby Showing Off Her Heels as She Heals

We all have obstacles to overcome no matter who we are. When you are, a healthy person faced with a challenge, think about how you feel when others want to help you. What if you are heavy set, bald or short and people are treating you differently from the rest of the family or community. Like you, the disabled person would rather not be pitied or shunned because of their disability. They would much rather be accepted for who they are.

Recognizing that the disabled person in the family has normal thoughts and feelings can go a long way. Just by asking questions, aiding, and putting yourself in their shoes can help all your lives in a positive, healthy way, and you might learn more about yourself in the process.

Remember to communicate with your caregivers and loved ones. We need to be the chief of staff of our own personal medical team. Become the expert of yourself and our illness.

My final thoughts are these 4 steps that patients can do to head in the right direction for pain relief. 1) Speak UP! You are your best advocate and have a right to timely and effective care. 2) Know your pain. Know the options available and educate yourself about available treatment options for your conditions. 3) Reach out and seek out. Bring a caregiver, relative or friend to your appointments so they can take notes and serve as an objective voice to your issues, accept assistance from others and investigate resources in your community or online. 4) Take a moment to listen to your body's response to stress and anxiety. Maintain healthy habits and stay active to the best of your ability. Make a habit of taking time each day for deep breathing exercises to help ease your pain.

For me, living life daily with chronic pain is improved creating an oasis environment. I pace my activities, keep a journal of what helps and doesn't. I keep items I use often accessible around the house. I do my daily stretching and relaxation techniques. And finally, I created a support system that is positive and uplifting.

I encourage each of you to become your own best advocate and seek the care that will be best for you and your health. Keep track of the things that are important to you physically, spiritually and mentally. The better you take care of yourself, the better others can help you.

BOOKS BY BARBY INGLE

- *Aunt Barby's Invisible, Endless Owie (co-author)*

- *From Wheels to Heals*

- *I'm Possible Book Project (co-author)*

- *Real Love; For Chronic Pain Patients and Their Partners (co-author)*

- *Remission Possible; Yours If You Choose to Accept It*

- *RSD In Me; A Patient and Caregivers Guide to Living with Reflex Sympathetic Dystrophy and Other Pain Diseases*

- *The Pain Code; Navigating the Minefield of the Health System*

- *The Pain Code; Journal (Supplement to The Pain Code Book)*

- *The Wisdom of Ingle; Fall Down and Get Up in Half a Day (co-author)*

Available everywhere books are sold!

Made in the USA
Coppell, TX
28 April 2022